This Patient Care Notebook Belongs to:

___

Nurse Life

DEDICATION

This book is dedicated to all the awesome nurses and front line workers out there!

You are my inspiration in producing books and I'm excited to help in the planning of your nursing care of patients around the world!

How to Use this Patient Care Notebook:

The purpose of this nurse shift report journal is to keep all your various patient reports all organized in one easy to find spot.

Here are some simple guidelines to follow so you can make the most of using this book:

1. The first "Patient Vital Signs" section is for you to write out all pertinent patient information, date of birth, diagnosis, vital signs, pain level...so you can go back there to be reminded of this info when you get ready to chart or give a report to the oncoming nurse.

2. Most ideas are inspired by something we have seen. Use the "Medical Progress Reporting" section to use as a reminder the date and time, what you observed, what the patient said, as you needed that information.

3. The "Physician Comments" section is for you to write out all the notes and information that the doctor has ordered for that patient, things to do, to keep an up to date record your journey of taking care of your patients while on your shift.

4. Finally, even more pages with "Additional Notes" sections so as to lay out your plan of keeping up with your patients, change of condition, pain relief and much more!

5. Whether you've just started as a new nurse or a seasoned pro...you will want this notebook to look back on and remember the things you've done for each patient under your care.

Patient Vital Signs Record Sheet

Name:	Notes/Comments:
Date of Birth:	
Diagnosis:	
Emergency Contact:	
Dr. Name/Number:	

Date/Time	Weight	Pulse	Blood Pressure	Temperature	Respirations	Pain Level 1-10	Initials

List Medication(s):

Medical Progress Reporting

Name/Medical Record #		Physician Notes/Comments
Date/Time	Medical Observation Notes	

Additional Notes:

Patient Vital Signs Record Sheet

Name:	Notes/Comments:
Date of Birth:	
Diagnosis:	
Emergency Contact:	
Dr. Name/Number:	

Date/Time	Weight	Pulse	Blood Pressure	Temperature	Respirations	Pain Level 1-10	Initials

List Medication(s):

Medical Progress Reporting

Name/Medical Record #		Physician Notes/Comments
Date/Time	Medical Observation Notes	

Additional Notes:

Nurse Life

Patient Vital Signs Record Sheet

Name:	Notes/Comments:
Date of Birth:	
Diagnosis:	
Emergency Contact:	
Dr. Name/Number:	

Date/Time	Weight	Pulse	Blood Pressure	Temperature	Respirations	Pain Level 1-10	Initials

List Medication(s):

Medical Progress Reporting

Name/Medical Record #		Physician Notes/Comments
Date/Time	Medical Observation Notes	

Additional Notes:

Patient Vital Signs Record Sheet

Name:	Notes/Comments:
Date of Birth:	
Diagnosis:	
Emergency Contact:	
Dr. Name/Number:	

Date/Time	Weight	Pulse	Blood Pressure	Temperature	Respirations	Pain Level 1-10	Initials

List Medication(s):

Medical Progress Reporting

Name/Medical Record #		Physician Notes/Comments
Date/Time	Medical Observation Notes	

Additional Notes:

Nurse Life

Patient Vital Signs Record Sheet

Name:	Notes/Comments:
Date of Birth:	
Diagnosis:	
Emergency Contact:	
Dr. Name/Number:	

Date/Time	Weight	Pulse	Blood Pressure	Temperature	Respirations	Pain Level 1-10	Initials

List Medication(s):

Medical Progress Reporting

Name/Medical Record #		Physician Notes/Comments
Date/Time	Medical Observation Notes	

Additional Notes:

Nurse Life

Patient Vital Signs Record Sheet

Name:	Notes/Comments:
Date of Birth:	
Diagnosis:	
Emergency Contact:	
Dr. Name/Number:	

Date/Time	Weight	Pulse	Blood Pressure	Temperature	Respirations	Pain Level 1-10	Initials

List Medication(s):

Medical Progress Reporting

Name/Medical Record #		Physician Notes/Comments
Date/Time	Medical Observation Notes	

Additional Notes:

Nurse Life

Patient Vital Signs Record Sheet

Name:	Notes/Comments:
Date of Birth:	
Diagnosis:	
Emergency Contact:	
Dr. Name/Number:	

Date/Time	Weight	Pulse	Blood Pressure	Temperature	Respirations	Pain Level 1-10	Initials

List Medication(s):

Medical Progress Reporting

Name/Medical Record #		Physician Notes/Comments
Date/Time	Medical Observation Notes	

Additional Notes:

Nurse Life

Patient Vital Signs Record Sheet

Name:	Notes/Comments:
Date of Birth:	
Diagnosis:	
Emergency Contact:	
Dr. Name/Number:	

Date/Time	Weight	Pulse	Blood Pressure	Temperature	Respirations	Pain Level 1-10	Initials

List Medication(s):

Medical Progress Reporting

Name/Medical Record #		Physician Notes/Comments
Date/Time	Medical Observation Notes	

Additional Notes:

Patient Vital Signs Record Sheet

Name:

Date of Birth:

Diagnosis:

Emergency Contact:

Notes/Comments:

Dr. Name/Number:

Date/Time	Weight	Pulse	Blood Pressure	Temperature	Respirations	Pain Level 1-10	Initials

List Medication(s):

Medical Progress Reporting

Name/Medical Record #		Physician Notes/Comments
Date/Time	Medical Observation Notes	

Additional Notes:

Nurse Life

Patient Vital Signs Record Sheet

Name:	Notes/Comments:
Date of Birth:	
Diagnosis:	
Emergency Contact:	
Dr. Name/Number:	

Date/Time	Weight	Pulse	Blood Pressure	Temperature	Respirations	Pain Level 1-10	Initials

List Medication(s):

Medical Progress Reporting

Name/Medical Record #

Date/Time	Medical Observation Notes	Physician Notes/Comments

Additional Notes:

Patient Vital Signs Record Sheet

Name:	Notes/Comments:
Date of Birth:	
Diagnosis:	
Emergency Contact:	
Dr. Name/Number:	

Date/Time	Weight	Pulse	Blood Pressure	Temperature	Respirations	Pain Level 1-10	Initials

List Medication(s):

Medical Progress Reporting

Name/Medical Record #		Physician Notes/Comments
Date/Time	Medical Observation Notes	

Additional Notes:

Nurse Life

Patient Vital Signs Record Sheet

Name:	Notes/Comments:
Date of Birth:	
Diagnosis:	
Emergency Contact:	
Dr. Name/Number:	

Date/Time	Weight	Pulse	Blood Pressure	Temperature	Respirations	Pain Level 1-10	Initials

List Medication(s):

Medical Progress Reporting

Name/Medical Record #		Physician Notes/Comments
Date/Time	Medical Observation Notes	

Additional Notes:

Patient Vital Signs Record Sheet

Name:	Notes/Comments:
Date of Birth:	
Diagnosis:	
Emergency Contact:	

Dr. Name/Number:

Date/Time	Weight	Pulse	Blood Pressure	Temperature	Respirations	Pain Level 1-10	Initials

List Medication(s):

Medical Progress Reporting

Name/Medical Record #		Physician Notes/Comments
Date/Time	Medical Observation Notes	

Additional Notes:

Nurse Life

Patient Vital Signs Record Sheet

Name:	Notes/Comments:
Date of Birth:	
Diagnosis:	
Emergency Contact:	
Dr. Name/Number:	

Date/Time	Weight	Pulse	Blood Pressure	Temperature	Respirations	Pain Level 1-10	Initials

List Medication(s):

Medical Progress Reporting

Name/Medical Record #		Physician Notes/Comments
Date/Time	Medical Observation Notes	

Additional Notes:

Nurse Life

Patient Vital Signs Record Sheet

Name:	Notes/Comments:
Date of Birth:	
Diagnosis:	
Emergency Contact:	
Dr. Name/Number:	

Date/Time	Weight	Pulse	Blood Pressure	Temperature	Respirations	Pain Level 1-10	Initials

List Medication(s):

Medical Progress Reporting

Name/Medical Record #		Physician Notes/Comments
Date/Time	Medical Observation Notes	

Additional Notes:

Nurse Life

Patient Vital Signs Record Sheet

Name:	Notes/Comments:
Date of Birth:	
Diagnosis:	
Emergency Contact:	

Dr. Name/Number:

Date/Time	Weight	Pulse	Blood Pressure	Temperature	Respirations	Pain Level 1-10	Initials

List Medication(s):

Medical Progress Reporting

Name/Medical Record #

Date/Time	Medical Observation Notes	Physician Notes/Comments

Additional Notes:

Patient Vital Signs Record Sheet

Name:	Notes/Comments:
Date of Birth:	
Diagnosis:	
Emergency Contact:	
Dr. Name/Number:	

Date/Time	Weight	Pulse	Blood Pressure	Temperature	Respirations	Pain Level 1-10	Initials

List Medication(s):

Medical Progress Reporting

Name/Medical Record #		Physician Notes/Comments
Date/Time	**Medical Observation Notes**	

Additional Notes:

Nurse Life

Patient Vital Signs Record Sheet

Name:	Notes/Comments:
Date of Birth:	
Diagnosis:	
Emergency Contact:	
Dr. Name/Number:	

Date/Time	Weight	Pulse	Blood Pressure	Temperature	Respirations	Pain Level 1-10	Initials

List Medication(s):

Medical Progress Reporting

Name/Medical Record #		Physician Notes/Comments
Date/Time	Medical Observation Notes	

Additional Notes:

Patient Vital Signs Record Sheet

Name:	Notes/Comments:
Date of Birth:	
Diagnosis:	
Emergency Contact:	
Dr. Name/Number:	

Date/Time	Weight	Pulse	Blood Pressure	Temperature	Respirations	Pain Level 1-10	Initials

List Medication(s):

Medical Progress Reporting

Name/Medical Record #		Physician Notes/Comments
Date/Time	Medical Observation Notes	

Additional Notes:

Patient Vital Signs Record Sheet

Name:	Notes/Comments:
Date of Birth:	
Diagnosis:	
Emergency Contact:	
Dr. Name/Number:	

Date/Time	Weight	Pulse	Blood Pressure	Temperature	Respirations	Pain Level 1-10	Initials

List Medication(s):

Medical Progress Reporting

Name/Medical Record #		Physician Notes/Comments
Date/Time	Medical Observation Notes	

Additional Notes:

Patient Vital Signs Record Sheet

Name:	Notes/Comments:
Date of Birth:	
Diagnosis:	
Emergency Contact:	
Dr. Name/Number:	

Date/Time	Weight	Pulse	Blood Pressure	Temperature	Respirations	Pain Level 1-10	Initials

List Medication(s):

Medical Progress Reporting

Name/Medical Record #		Physician Notes/Comments
Date/Time	Medical Observation Notes	

Additional Notes:

Nurse Life

Patient Vital Signs Record Sheet

Name:	Notes/Comments:
Date of Birth:	
Diagnosis:	
Emergency Contact:	
Dr. Name/Number:	

Date/Time	Weight	Pulse	Blood Pressure	Temperature	Respirations	Pain Level 1-10	Initials

List Medication(s):

Medical Progress Reporting

Name/Medical Record #		Physician Notes/Comments
Date/Time	Medical Observation Notes	

Additional Notes:

Nurse Life

Patient Vital Signs Record Sheet

Name:	Notes/Comments:
Date of Birth:	
Diagnosis:	
Emergency Contact:	
Dr. Name/Number:	

Date/Time	Weight	Pulse	Blood Pressure	Temperature	Respirations	Pain Level 1-10	Initials

List Medication(s):

Medical Progress Reporting

Name/Medical Record #		Physician Notes/Comments
Date/Time	Medical Observation Notes	

Additional Notes:

Nurse Life

Patient Vital Signs Record Sheet

Name:	Notes/Comments:
Date of Birth:	
Diagnosis:	
Emergency Contact:	

Dr. Name/Number:

Date/Time	Weight	Pulse	Blood Pressure	Temperature	Respirations	Pain Level 1-10	Initials

List Medication(s):

Medical Progress Reporting

Name/Medical Record #

Date/Time	Medical Observation Notes	Physician Notes/Comments

Additional Notes:

Nurse Life

Patient Vital Signs Record Sheet

Name:	Notes/Comments:
Date of Birth:	
Diagnosis:	
Emergency Contact:	
Dr. Name/Number:	

Date/Time	Weight	Pulse	Blood Pressure	Temperature	Respirations	Pain Level 1-10	Initials

List Medication(s):

Medical Progress Reporting

Name/Medical Record #		Physician Notes/Comments
Date/Time	Medical Observation Notes	

Additional Notes:

Nurse Life

Patient Vital Signs Record Sheet

Name:	Notes/Comments:
Date of Birth:	
Diagnosis:	
Emergency Contact:	
Dr. Name/Number:	

Date/Time	Weight	Pulse	Blood Pressure	Temperature	Respirations	Pain Level 1-10	Initials

List Medication(s):

Medical Progress Reporting

Name/Medical Record #		Physician Notes/Comments
Date/Time	Medical Observation Notes	

Additional Notes:

Nurse Life

Patient Vital Signs Record Sheet

Name:	Notes/Comments:
Date of Birth:	
Diagnosis:	
Emergency Contact:	
Dr. Name/Number:	

Date/Time	Weight	Pulse	Blood Pressure	Temperature	Respirations	Pain Level 1-10	Initials

List Medication(s):

Medical Progress Reporting

Name/Medical Record #		Physician Notes/Comments
Date/Time	Medical Observation Notes	

Additional Notes:

Nurse Life

Patient Vital Signs Record Sheet

Name:

Date of Birth:

Diagnosis:

Emergency Contact:

Notes/Comments:

Dr. Name/Number:

Date/Time	Weight	Pulse	Blood Pressure	Temperature	Respirations	Pain Level 1-10	Initials

List Medication(s):

Medical Progress Reporting

Name/Medical Record #		Physician Notes/Comments
Date/Time	Medical Observation Notes	

Additional Notes:

Nurse Life

Patient Vital Signs Record Sheet

Name:	Notes/Comments:
Date of Birth:	
Diagnosis:	
Emergency Contact:	
Dr. Name/Number:	

Date/Time	Weight	Pulse	Blood Pressure	Temperature	Respirations	Pain Level 1-10	Initials

List Medication(s):

Medical Progress Reporting

Name/Medical Record #

Date/Time	Medical Observation Notes	Physician Notes/Comments

Additional Notes:

Nurse Life

Patient Vital Signs Record Sheet

Name:	Notes/Comments:
Date of Birth:	
Diagnosis:	
Emergency Contact:	
Dr. Name/Number:	

Date/Time	Weight	Pulse	Blood Pressure	Temperature	Respirations	Pain Level 1-10	Initials

List Medication(s):

Medical Progress Reporting

Name/Medical Record #		Physician Notes/Comments
Date/Time	Medical Observation Notes	

Additional Notes:

Nurse Life

Patient Vital Signs Record Sheet

Name:	Notes/Comments:
Date of Birth:	
Diagnosis:	
Emergency Contact:	
Dr. Name/Number:	

Date/Time	Weight	Pulse	Blood Pressure	Temperature	Respirations	Pain Level 1-10	Initials

List Medication(s):

Medical Progress Reporting

Name/Medical Record #		Physician Notes/Comments
Date/Time	Medical Observation Notes	
Additional Notes:		

Patient Vital Signs Record Sheet

Name:	Notes/Comments:
Date of Birth:	
Diagnosis:	
Emergency Contact:	
Dr. Name/Number:	

Date/Time	Weight	Pulse	Blood Pressure	Temperature	Respirations	Pain Level 1-10	Initials

List Medication(s):

Medical Progress Reporting

Name/Medical Record #		Physician Notes/Comments
Date/Time	Medical Observation Notes	

Additional Notes:

Patient Vital Signs Record Sheet

Name:	Notes/Comments:
Date of Birth:	
Diagnosis:	
Emergency Contact:	
Dr. Name/Number:	

Date/Time	Weight	Pulse	Blood Pressure	Temperature	Respirations	Pain Level 1-10	Initials

List Medication(s):

Medical Progress Reporting

Name/Medical Record #		Physician Notes/Comments
Date/Time	Medical Observation Notes	

Additional Notes:

Nurse Life

Patient Vital Signs Record Sheet

Name:

Date of Birth:

Diagnosis:

Emergency Contact:

Notes/Comments:

Dr. Name/Number:

Date/Time	Weight	Pulse	Blood Pressure	Temperature	Respirations	Pain Level 1-10	Initials

List Medication(s):

Medical Progress Reporting

Name/Medical Record #

Date/Time	Medical Observation Notes	Physician Notes/Comments

Additional Notes:

Nurse Life

Patient Vital Signs Record Sheet

Name:	Notes/Comments:
Date of Birth:	
Diagnosis:	
Emergency Contact:	
Dr. Name/Number:	

Date/Time	Weight	Pulse	Blood Pressure	Temperature	Respirations	Pain Level 1-10	Initials

List Medication(s):

Medical Progress Reporting

Name/Medical Record #		Physician Notes/Comments
Date/Time	Medical Observation Notes	

Additional Notes:

Nurse Life

Patient Vital Signs Record Sheet

Name:	Notes/Comments:
Date of Birth:	
Diagnosis:	
Emergency Contact:	

Dr. Name/Number:

Date/Time	Weight	Pulse	Blood Pressure	Temperature	Respirations	Pain Level 1-10	Initials

List Medication(s):

Medical Progress Reporting

Name/Medical Record #		Physician Notes/Comments
Date/Time	Medical Observation Notes	

Additional Notes:

Nurse Life

Patient Vital Signs Record Sheet

Name:	Notes/Comments:
Date of Birth:	
Diagnosis:	
Emergency Contact:	
Dr. Name/Number:	

Date/Time	Weight	Pulse	Blood Pressure	Temperature	Respirations	Pain Level 1-10	Initials

List Medication(s):

Medical Progress Reporting

Name/Medical Record #		Physician Notes/Comments
Date/Time	Medical Observation Notes	

Additional Notes:

Nurse Life

Patient Vital Signs Record Sheet

Name:	Notes/Comments:
Date of Birth:	
Diagnosis:	
Emergency Contact:	
Dr. Name/Number:	

Date/Time	Weight	Pulse	Blood Pressure	Temperature	Respirations	Pain Level 1-10	Initials

List Medication(s):

Medical Progress Reporting

Name/Medical Record #

Date/Time	Medical Observation Notes	Physician Notes/Comments

Additional Notes:

Nurse Life

Patient Vital Signs Record Sheet

Name:	Notes/Comments:
Date of Birth:	
Diagnosis:	
Emergency Contact:	
Dr. Name/Number:	

Date/Time	Weight	Pulse	Blood Pressure	Temperature	Respirations	Pain Level 1-10	Initials

List Medication(s):

Medical Progress Reporting

Name/Medical Record #		
Date/Time	Medical Observation Notes	Physician Notes/Comments

Additional Notes:

Nurse Life

Patient Vital Signs Record Sheet

Name:	Notes/Comments:
Date of Birth:	
Diagnosis:	
Emergency Contact:	
Dr. Name/Number:	

Date/Time	Weight	Pulse	Blood Pressure	Temperature	Respirations	Pain Level 1-10	Initials

List Medication(s):

Medical Progress Reporting

Name/Medical Record #

Date/Time	Medical Observation Notes	Physician Notes/Comments

Additional Notes:

Patient Vital Signs Record Sheet

Name:	Notes/Comments:
Date of Birth:	
Diagnosis:	
Emergency Contact:	

Dr. Name/Number:

Date/Time	Weight	Pulse	Blood Pressure	Temperature	Respirations	Pain Level 1-10	Initials

List Medication(s):

Medical Progress Reporting

Name/Medical Record #		Physician Notes/Comments
Date/Time	Medical Observation Notes	

Additional Notes:

Nurse Life

Patient Vital Signs Record Sheet

Name:	Notes/Comments:
Date of Birth:	
Diagnosis:	
Emergency Contact:	

Dr. Name/Number:

Date/Time	Weight	Pulse	Blood Pressure	Temperature	Respirations	Pain Level 1-10	Initials

List Medication(s):

Medical Progress Reporting

Name/Medical Record #		Physician Notes/Comments
Date/Time	Medical Observation Notes	

Additional Notes:

Nurse Life

Patient Vital Signs Record Sheet

Name:	Notes/Comments:
Date of Birth:	
Diagnosis:	
Emergency Contact:	
Dr. Name/Number:	

Date/Time	Weight	Pulse	Blood Pressure	Temperature	Respirations	Pain Level 1-10	Initials

List Medication(s):

Medical Progress Reporting

Name/Medical Record #		Physician Notes/Comments
Date/Time	Medical Observation Notes	

Additional Notes:

Patient Vital Signs Record Sheet

Name:	Notes/Comments:
Date of Birth:	
Diagnosis:	
Emergency Contact:	
Dr. Name/Number:	

Date/Time	Weight	Pulse	Blood Pressure	Temperature	Respirations	Pain Level 1-10	Initials

List Medication(s):

Medical Progress Reporting

Name/Medical Record #		Physician Notes/Comments
Date/Time	Medical Observation Notes	

Additional Notes:

Patient Vital Signs Record Sheet

Name:	Notes/Comments:
Date of Birth:	
Diagnosis:	
Emergency Contact:	
Dr. Name/Number:	

Date/Time	Weight	Pulse	Blood Pressure	Temperature	Respirations	Pain Level 1-10	Initials

List Medication(s):

Medical Progress Reporting

Name/Medical Record #

Date/Time	Medical Observation Notes	Physician Notes/Comments

Additional Notes:

Nurse Life

Patient Vital Signs Record Sheet

Name:

Date of Birth:

Diagnosis:

Emergency Contact:

Notes/Comments:

Dr. Name/Number:

Date/Time	Weight	Pulse	Blood Pressure	Temperature	Respirations	Pain Level 1-10	Initials

List Medication(s):

Medical Progress Reporting

Name/Medical Record #		Physician Notes/Comments
Date/Time	Medical Observation Notes	

Additional Notes:

Nurse Life

Patient Vital Signs Record Sheet

Name:	Notes/Comments:
Date of Birth:	
Diagnosis:	
Emergency Contact:	
Dr. Name/Number:	

Date/Time	Weight	Pulse	Blood Pressure	Temperature	Respirations	Pain Level 1-10	Initials

List Medication(s):

Medical Progress Reporting

Name/Medical Record #		Physician Notes/Comments
Date/Time	Medical Observation Notes	

Additional Notes:

Nurse Life

Patient Vital Signs Record Sheet

Name:	Notes/Comments:
Date of Birth:	
Diagnosis:	
Emergency Contact:	
Dr. Name/Number:	

Date/Time	Weight	Pulse	Blood Pressure	Temperature	Respirations	Pain Level 1-10	Initials

List Medication(s):

Medical Progress Reporting

Name/Medical Record #		Physician Notes/Comments
Date/Time	Medical Observation Notes	

Additional Notes:

Patient Vital Signs Record Sheet

Name:	Notes/Comments:
Date of Birth:	
Diagnosis:	
Emergency Contact:	
Dr. Name/Number:	

Date/Time	Weight	Pulse	Blood Pressure	Temperature	Respirations	Pain Level 1-10	Initials

List Medication(s):

Medical Progress Reporting

Name/Medical Record #		Physician Notes/Comments
Date/Time	Medical Observation Notes	

Additional Notes:

Nurse Life

Patient Vital Signs Record Sheet

Name:	Notes/Comments:
Date of Birth:	
Diagnosis:	
Emergency Contact:	
Dr. Name/Number:	

Date/Time	Weight	Pulse	Blood Pressure	Temperature	Respirations	Pain Level 1-10	Initials

List Medication(s):

Medical Progress Reporting

Name/Medical Record #		Physician Notes/Comments
Date/Time	Medical Observation Notes	

Additional Notes:

Nurse Life

Patient Vital Signs Record Sheet

Name:	Notes/Comments:
Date of Birth:	
Diagnosis:	
Emergency Contact:	
Dr. Name/Number:	

Date/Time	Weight	Pulse	Blood Pressure	Temperature	Respirations	Pain Level 1-10	Initials

List Medication(s):

Medical Progress Reporting

Name/Medical Record #		Physician Notes/Comments
Date/Time	Medical Observation Notes	

Additional Notes:

Nurse Life

Patient Vital Signs Record Sheet

Name:	Notes/Comments:
Date of Birth:	
Diagnosis:	
Emergency Contact:	
Dr. Name/Number:	

Date/Time	Weight	Pulse	Blood Pressure	Temperature	Respirations	Pain Level 1-10	Initials

List Medication(s):

Medical Progress Reporting

Name/Medical Record #		Physician Notes/Comments
Date/Time	Medical Observation Notes	

Additional Notes:

Nurse Life

Patient Vital Signs Record Sheet

Name:	Notes/Comments:
Date of Birth:	
Diagnosis:	
Emergency Contact:	
Dr. Name/Number:	

Date/Time	Weight	Pulse	Blood Pressure	Temperature	Respirations	Pain Level 1-10	Initials

List Medication(s):

Medical Progress Reporting

Name/Medical Record #		Physician Notes/Comments
Date/Time	Medical Observation Notes	

Additional Notes:

Nurse Life

Patient Vital Signs Record Sheet

Name:	Notes/Comments:
Date of Birth:	
Diagnosis:	
Emergency Contact:	
Dr. Name/Number:	

Date/Time	Weight	Pulse	Blood Pressure	Temperature	Respirations	Pain Level 1-10	Initials

List Medication(s):

Medical Progress Reporting

Name/Medical Record #		Physician Notes/Comments
Date/Time	Medical Observation Notes	

Additional Notes:

Patient Vital Signs Record Sheet

Name:	Notes/Comments:
Date of Birth:	
Diagnosis:	
Emergency Contact:	
Dr. Name/Number:	

Date/Time	Weight	Pulse	Blood Pressure	Temperature	Respirations	Pain Level 1-10	Initials

List Medication(s):

Milton Keynes UK
Ingram Content Group UK Ltd.
UKHW030036071123
432059UK00014B/471

THE HAMLYN DIET

Michelle Bonnic

Contents

1. INTRODUCTION 1
2. QUESADILLAS 7
3. STUFFED COURGETTES 9
4. FRITTATA WITH ASPARAGUS 11
5. FALAFEL 13
6. AUBERGINE LIQUIFIES 17
7. FRITTERS OF SWEETCORN 19
8. AVOCADO AND TOMATO TOSTADOS 23
9. MOZZARELLA AND SPINACH PANCAKES 27
10. FLORENTINE EGGS 31
11. ROSTIS 33
12. BOATS 37
13. BRUSCHETTA 39
14. PITAS 41
15. BAKED BRIE 43
16. CROSTINI 45

17. POACHED EGGS 49
18. OMELETTE 51
19. BEAN BURGERS 53
20. FILLED PEPPERS 57
21. CIABATTA TOAST WITH VEGETABLES 59
22. SOUP 1 61
23. SOUP 2 63
24. SOUP 3 67
25. SOUP 4 71
26. SOUP 5 73
27. GREEN GAZPACHO 75
28. SPICY LENTILS SOUP 79
29. TUSCAN BEAN AND TRUFFLES SOUP 83
30. GOAT CHEESE AND BEETS SALAD 85
31. PUMPKIN AND APPLES SOUP 87
32. SPICY SOYA AND NOODLES SALAD 91
33. BULGUR SALAD 93
34. QUINOA AND TOMATOES SALAD 95
35. PANZANELLA 99
36. CHICKPEAS SALAD 101

37. QUINOA RISOTTO 103
38. PIE WITH SPINACH 105
39. PILAU 109
40. EGGS WITH A RANCH FLAVOR 111
41. POTATO GNOCCHI 113
42. NAAN 115
43. COURGETTE AND FETA FRITTERS 117
44. RISOTTO WITH TOMATOES 121
45. CHEESE AND SPINACH CALZONE 123
46. PASTA 127
47. TAGINE DE LEGUMES 129
48. PEPPER PIZZA 133
49. SPAGHETTI 135
50. ARRABBIATA 139
51. MEDITERRANEAN BEANS 141
52. GRATIN 143

Chapter One

INTRODUCTION

This book introduces a unique and flexible method to meal planning for busy cooks, allowing you to select the recipe option that best fits your time constraints. There are 200 recipes inside that will inspire and motivate you to cook every day of the year.

All of the recipes take no more than 30 minutes to prepare. Some can be completed in as little as 20 minutes, and many can be completed in as little as 10 minutes.

Every page includes a main recipe as well as a quick-fix version or a fancier variation if you have a little more time. Whatever you choose, there's a vast selection of super-fast dishes to get you through the week.

Recipes for vegetarians

It is well known that a diet rich in fresh vegetables, legumes, and wholegrains is healthy. With the understanding that a high-protein diet can be harmful to one's health, and with such a broad variety of delicious, seasonal vegetables readily available, it's easy to see why so many people prefer to adopt a vegetarian or 'flexitarian' diet.

The key to a well-balanced vegetarian diet is to consume a variety of wholegrains (brown rice, barley, corn, oats, millet, and buckwheat are all good choices), wholegrain-based foods (wholemeal breads, pastas, and cereals), protein-rich pulses, lentils, nuts, and eggs, as well as plenty of fresh fruit and vegetables. Caffeinated drinks, alcohol, and sweet snacks should be used in moderation, as should dairy products (such as butter, cheese, cream, milk, and yoghurt) or non-dairy equivalents.

Complex carbohydrates are necessary for a healthy diet and provide energy. Dietary fiber permits the energy from the natural sugars it contains to be released gradually, as opposed to processed carbohydrates, which are quickly absorbed by the body and can deplete energy levels. Foods prepared with the whole grain, such as wholemeal bread and wholewheat pasta, as well as brown rice, barley, corn, buckwheat, dry beans, and bananas, are high in complex carbs.

Fibre is essential for passing food through the bowels, preventing digestive issues and lowering the risk of bowel cancer. A healthy vegetarian diet will be high in fibre. Because high-fibre foods like beans and peas, brassica family veggies (such as cabbage, broccoli, and brussels sprouts), oats, and wholegrain wheat can help lower blood cholesterol, it's a good idea to include them in most of your meals.

Protein is necessary for tissue healing, cell growth, and reproduction, particularly in youngsters and pregnant women. However, we don't need a lot of protein in our diet, and it's absolutely possible to get all of the protein we need from non-animal sources. Nuts and seeds, pulses, soy products, peas, beans, chickpeas, and lentils are all good sources of vegetarian protein.

Techniques and suggestions

Using condiments, seasonings, herbs, and spices may greatly enhance your eating experience, allowing you to make and eat a diverse range of flavors, colors, and textures. Before you begin your journey through the wide and fascinating world of vegetarian cooking, stock up on supplies. Most supermarkets will have everything you need, but for more unique products and produce, try ethnic stores and greengrocers.

When it comes to making vegetarian meals, having a well-equipped kitchen will save you a lot of time. A few decent saucepans of various sizes, a frying pan, and a wok are all necessary, and a good-quality pestle and mortar will come in handy. Salad washing can be sped up using a salad spinner, and precise kitchen scales will assure consistent results. For quick and easy blending and processing, a food processor is a necessary.

Stock up on pantry essentials.

Having a range of dried pasta forms on hand is a good idea — linguini, spaghetti, pappardelle, fusilli, penne, and orzo should cover most recipes. Rice (basmati, brown, jasmine, risotto, and paella), bulgar wheat, couscous, polenta, and quinoa are all excellent staples that may be utilized in a variety of ways to make delicious, simple meals. For sauce bases and crumble toppings, plain flour is a requirement. Gram flour can be used to make a spicy batter that can be used to make a variety of crispy veggie fritters.

Puy lentils, split red lentils, and yellow split peas are quick-cooking pulses that don't need to be soaked for long periods of time, and canned pulses and beans are great for quick, last-minute dinners. Kidney beans, chickpeas, black-eyed beans, cannellini beans, and butter beans are all nice to have on hand.

Nuts and seeds are nutritious, healthful, and delicious additions to a variety of recipes, from salads to stir-fries. Sunflower seeds, sesame seeds, cashew nuts, almonds, pistachios, and walnuts are all healthy vegetarian additions.

Canned tomatoes and passata are a great standby for preparing quick sauces, curries, and stews because they're packed with flavor and color.

Stir-frying and general-purpose cooking are made easier with good-quality olive oil, sunflower and vegetable oils, and toasted sesame seed oil. For quick salad dressings and sauces, red wine, white wine, balsamic, cider, and rice wine vinegars are essential.

Flavourings

You can never have enough dried herbs and spices in your pantry to experiment with different flavors. The list goes on and on, but remember to buy in modest quantities and use within three months for the best flavor. A good stock of dried herbs (basil, thyme, oregano, tarragon, rosemary, and parsley are good places to start), whole spices (cumin seeds, coriander seeds, black mustard seeds, cloves, cardamom pods, and cinnamon sticks), and ground spices (cumin, cinnamon, coriander, chili powder, paprika, and turmeric) will give your dishes a lot of depth. Fresh black peppercorns and sea salt are also essential.

To add instant flavor to your dishes, stock up on a variety of sauces and condiments. You'll use soy sauce, sweet chili sauce, tabasco sauce, and Worcestershire sauce over and over again. Honey and maple syrup are versatile sweeteners that can be used in both sweet and savory dishes.

Food that is fresh

Maintaining a well-stocked refrigerator will allow you to prepare healthy and delectable vegetarian meals in a matter of minutes. To reduce waste, buy fresh vegetables on a regular basis and only buy what you know you'll utilize. Fresh pasta, tofu, cheese, butter, milk, cream, and eggs are always welcome additions to the refrigerator. Lemons, limes, red chillies, fresh ginger, spring onions, and fresh herbs are other good complements to quick dinners.

Fruit and vegetables that are in season and, if possible, farmed locally should be purchased. The quality and flavor will be significantly greater to those cultivated out of season or that have traveled hundreds of miles to reach supermarket shelves. Garlic, onions, potatoes, shallots, carrots and other root vegetables, as well as most fruits, will stay in the pantry for a few days.

Chapter Two

QUESADILLAS

Quesadillas a la minute

4 servings

10 minutes total cooking time

refried beans, 200 g (7 oz)

8 flour tortillas, soft

25 g (1 oz) drained and cut jalapeo pepper slices

1 large deseeded and diced tomato

150 g (5 oz) grated cheddar cheese

2 sliced spring onions

1 tablespoon fresh coriander, freshly chopped (optional)

Sour cream, 100 mL (312 fl oz), to serve (optional)

4 of the tortillas should be covered in refried beans. If using, garnish with jalapeo slices, diced tomato, grated cheese,

spring onions, and chopped coriander. To make 4 quesadillas, cover each one with another tortilla.

In a large ridged griddle pan heated over medium-high heat, toast the quesadillas one at a time for 30–60 seconds on each side, until gently browned and the cheese inside has melted.

If adding soured cream, cut the quesadillas in quarters and serve immediately.

Spread refried beans over all 8 tortillas, then top with jalapeo slices, 2 large diced tomatoes, 1 cored, deseeded and chopped red pepper, and sliced spring onion for spicy bean burritos. Tuck the ends in and roll each tortilla securely, then place in an ovenproof dish that fits snugly. Over the tortillas, pour a 300 g (10 oz) container of hot mexican salsa, then dot with small spoonfuls of soured cream and sprinkle with cheese. Cook for 20–25 minutes at 220°C (425°F), gas mark 7 in a preheated oven until hot and bubbling. If used, top with shredded iceberg lettuce and chopped coriander. Cooking time is 30 minutes total.

Chapter Three

STUFFED COURGETTES

4 servings

30 minutes total cooking time

courgettes (four)

175 g (6 oz) diced plum tomatoes

210 g (7 oz) grated mozzarella cheese

2 tblsp basil leaves, shredded

25 g (1 oz) grated parmesan cheese

seasoning with salt and pepper

Cut the courgettes in half horizontally and scoop out the middles, reserving the flesh.

Place the courgette halves, cut side up, in a roasting tin and bake for 10 minutes at 200°C (400°F), gas mark 6.

In the meantime, cut the saved courgette flesh and combine it with chopped tomatoes, grated mozzarella, and basil in a mixing bowl. Season with salt and pepper to taste.

Remove the courgette halves from the oven and fill each half with the filling.

Return to the oven for 15 minutes, or until golden, then top with grated parmesan.

Use a vegetable peeler to thinly slice 4 courgettes lengthwise for griddled courgettes with mozzarella. Toss the courgettes in 2 tablespoons olive oil and fry for 2–3 minutes on both sides on a prepared hot griddle pan, until griddle marks appear. 210 g (7 oz) torn mozzarella cheese and 6–8 torn basil leaves are served on top. Add a drizzle of olive oil, a squeeze of lemon juice, and a pinch of black pepper. Cooking time is 20 minutes total.

Chapter Four

FRITTATA WITH ASPARAGUS

4 servings

30 minutes total cooking time

Asparagus, 400 g (13 oz)

2 tablespoons extra virgin olive oil

a dozen big eggs

50 g (2 oz) grated parmesan cheese

1 tablespoon oregano, chopped

seasoning with salt and pepper

Remove and discard the woody ends of the asparagus. 1 tablespoon olive oil toss the spears in.

Heat a griddle pan over high heat and fry the asparagus for 4–5 minutes, or until it begins to sear. Asparagus spears should be cut into thirds.

In a large mixing bowl, whisk together the eggs, grated parmesan, oregano, and a pinch of salt and pepper. Toss in the asparagus.

In a flameproof, nonstick frying pan, heat the remaining oil. Pour the mixture into the pan and simmer over low heat for 8–10 minutes, tipping the pan occasionally to allow the runny egg to reach the sides and cook evenly.

Cook for an additional 4–5 minutes under a preheated hot grill, or until browned on top.

Serve the frittata right away by turning it out onto a cutting board and cutting it into wedges.

Toss 450 g (112 oz) trimmed asparagus in 2 tablespoons olive oil for griddled asparagus. Cook the asparagus for 4–5 minutes, stirring once, on a hot griddle pan. Drizzle with olive oil and parmesan cheese shavings before serving. Cooking time is 10 minutes total.

Chapter Five

FALAFEL

4 servings

15-minute total cooking time

400 g (13 oz) rinsed and drained chickpeas

1 finely diced onion

2 chopped garlic cloves

3 tblsp. parsley, chopped

1 teaspoon coriander powder

1 teaspoon cumin powder

2 tablespoons all-purpose flour

2–3 tblsp. oil (vegetable)

seasoning with salt and pepper

12 iceberg lettuce leaves, shredded

sauce with a kick

Tomato purée, 100 g (312 oz)

12–1 teaspoon harissa paste, depending on personal preference

2 smashed garlic cloves

1 tsp lemon extract

2 fl oz water, 50 ml

1 tablespoon parsley, chopped

To prepare the sauce, combine all of the ingredients in a small pot and cook for 10 minutes, stirring occasionally.

Meanwhile, in a large mixing bowl, mash together all of the falafel ingredients except the oil using a fork. Season with salt and pepper to taste. Alternatively, whizz the ingredients until smooth in a food processor. Form the mixture into tiny balls with damp palms and flatten gently.

In a frying pan, heat the vegetable oil and cook the falafel for 5–7 minutes, flipping once, until brown on all sides.

Serve with the spicy sauce on the lettuce.

Make the falafel as directed for falafel with spicy sauce and tabbouleh salad. Meanwhile, in a heatproof bowl, combine 250 g (8 oz) couscous and just cover with boiling water. Allow for a 10-minute rest period. With a fork, fluff the couscous, then add 2 tablespoons chopped mint, parsley, and chives,

3 diced tomatoes, and 12 sliced cucumber. Serve with falafel and hummus that has already been cooked. Cooking time is 20 minutes total.

Chapter Six

AUBERGINE LIQUIFIES

4 servings

30 minutes total cooking time

2 aubergines, cut in half lengthwise

4 tablespoons extra virgin olive oil

4 sliced tomatoes

200 g (7 oz) sliced mozzarella cheese

a smidgeononononononononononononon

2 tablespoons pine nuts, roasted

Pepper

To serve, a crisp green salad

Place the aubergine halves on a baking sheet, brush with olive oil, and bake for 20 minutes until softened in a preheated oven at 200°C (400°F), gas mark 6.

Remove the aubergine from the oven, top with tomato slices, and bake for an additional 5 minutes, or until the cheese has melted.

Season with pepper and serve with a crisp green salad strewn with basil leaves and pine nuts.

Cook 400 g (13 oz) pasta shapes of your choice until 'al dente' in a saucepan of boiling water according to the package instructions for aubergine & goats' cheese pasta. In a separate frying pan, heat 1 tablespoon olive oil and sauté 1 chopped onion and 2 sliced garlic cloves for 3–4 minutes. Cook for another 4–5 minutes after adding 1 chopped aubergine. Simmer for 3–4 minutes after adding a 400 g (13 oz) diced tomato can. Drain the pasta and add 100 g (312 oz) crumbled goats' cheese and a small handful of torn basil leaves to the sauce, stirring thoroughly. Cooking time is 20 minutes total.

Chapter Seven

FRITTERS OF SWEETCORN

4 servings

Cooking time total: 20 minutes

Sweetcorn, 275 g (9 oz) in a can

ordinary flour, 65 g (212 oz)

1 teaspoon powdered baking soda

1 beaten egg

12 red peppers, de-seeded, cored, and finely chopped

1 deseeded and coarsely chopped tiny red chili

6 tablespoons fresh coriander, chopped

2 tblsp. vegetable oil 1 tblsp. pepper

Salsa

1 tablespoon extra virgin olive oil

2 finely sliced tomatoes

12 coarsely chopped tiny red chillies

1 tablespoon light brown sugar, soft

2 tblsp fresh coriander, chopped

Drain the sweetcorn and blitz half of the kernels till practically smooth in a food processor. Stir in the remaining entire sweetcorn in a mixing basin. Combine the flour and baking powder in a sifter. Season with plenty of pepper and stir in the egg, red pepper, chili, and coriander.

In a large, heavy-bottomed nonstick frying pan, heat the oil over medium-high heat and add 4 spoonfuls of the mixture. Cook for 1 minute on each side, or until golden brown. Using a fish slice, remove the fish, drain on kitchen paper, and keep warm. Cook the rest of the mixture in the same manner (to make 8 fritters in total).

Meanwhile, combine all of the salsa ingredients in a serving bowl, season with pepper, and set aside.

Warm fritters are served with salsa on the side.

Make a 150 g (5 oz) packet pancake batter mix according to package directions, then add 8 tablespoons drained canned sweetcorn and 3 tablespoons chopped fresh coriander to make sweetcorn pancakes. Season to taste. In a frying pan over medium-high heat, heat a little vegetable oil, pour in a quarter of the mixture, and cook for 1 minute, then flip and cook for a few seconds on the other side. Cook the remaining mixture in the same manner as the first. If desired, top the pancakes with store-bought tomato salsa and a few rocket leaves. Cooking time is 10 minutes total.

Chapter Eight

AVOCADO AND TOMATO TOSTADOS

4 servings

10 minutes total cooking time

4 tortillas de maz

1 tablespoon oil (vegetable)

2 peeled and stoned avocados

2 fl ounce crème fraîche 50 ml

lime juice (about 2–3 teaspoons)

4 chopped tomatoes

1 tablespoon red onion, finely chopped

1 tbsp olive oil (extra virgin)

a handful of chopped fresh coriander, plus more to serve (optional)

seasoning with salt and pepper

Stamp out rounds from the tortillas with a 5 cm (2 inch) biscuit cutter; alternately, cut them into wedges. Brush them with vegetable oil, then set them on a baking sheet under a hot grill for 1 minute on each side, or until crisp. Allow to cool.

Meanwhile, in a food processor, puree the avocado flesh and crème fraîche until smooth. Season with 1 tablespoon lime juice and salt and pepper to taste. Toss the tomatoes, onion, and olive oil together, season with salt and pepper, then stir in the coriander.

Spread a little amount of the avocado mixture on each tortilla round, then top with tomato salsa and additional coriander, if desired.

In a saucepan, heat 1 tablespoon olive oil, add 1 finely chopped onion, and simmer for 5 minutes, or until softened, for tomato and tortilla soup. Stir in three finely sliced garlic cloves around the pan. 2 tsp chipotle purée, 400 g (13 oz) diced tomatoes, 1 tsp brown sugar, and a pinch of dried oregano 1 litre (134 quarts) vegetable stock, brought to a boil, then reduced to a low heat and left to simmer for 10 minutes. Whizz everything together in a stick blender until creamy, then season to taste. 2 corn tortillas, sliced into thin strips Heat 1 tablespoon vegetable oil in a large frying pan and cook the tortillas for 1–2 minutes, until golden and crisp. To serve, ladle the soup into bowls. 1 avocado, 50 g (2 oz) crumbled feta, crisp tortillas, and a handful of chopped fresh coriander are served on top. Cooking time is 30 minutes total.

Chapter Nine

MOZZARELLA AND SPINACH PANCAKES

4 servings

Cooking time total: 20 minutes

ordinary flour, 125 g (4 oz)

a grain of salt

two eggs

75 ml (3 fl oz) water and 200 ml (7 fl oz) milk

50 g (2 oz) melted butter

infant spinach leaves, 200 g (7 oz)

4 sliced tomatoes

400 g (13 oz) sliced mozzarella cheese

2 tblsp parmesan cheese, grated

In a large mixing basin, sift together the flour and salt. In the center, make a well and crack the eggs into it. Mix the eggs into the flour, then whisk in a little bit of the milk and water while continuing to whisk.

Half of the melted butter should be whisked into the pancake mixture, and the rest should be used to grease a frying pan. To remove any excess, wipe the pan with kitchen paper.

Pour about 2 teaspoons of batter into the pan and swirl to coat the bottom completely. Check that the pancake is cooked bottom after 1 minute, and then flip it over to cook the other side for a few seconds more.

Half of the pancake should be garnished with spinach leaves, sliced tomatoes, and sliced mozzarella. Fold and lightly press the second half of the pancake over the filled side. Keep warm by transferring the filled pancake to an ovenproof dish.

Rep with the rest of the ingredients. Sprinkle the grated parmesan over the pancakes and cook them briefly on a prepared hot grill until golden. Serve right away.

Layer 100 g (312 oz) spinach leaves with 400 g (13 oz) sliced mozzarella cheese, 2 thinly sliced beefsteak tomatoes, and 10–12 basil leaves on a big dish for a mozzarella & spinach salad. Drizzle with 3 tablespoons extra virgin olive oil and 1 tablespoon balsamic vinegar, then top with 2 teaspoons minced oregano and 2 tablespoons toasted pine nuts. Cooking time is 10 minutes total.

Serves 4 Bocconcini with fresh pesto aoli

Cooking time total: 20 minutes

fresh white breadcrumbs, 100 g (312 oz)

1 lemon zest, finely grated

a good sprinkling of chilli flakes

2 tblsp. dried thyme leaves

ordinary flour, 50 g (2 oz)

2 big beaten eggs

bocconcini (baby mozzarella balls) 300 g (10 oz), drained

Deep-frying oil made from vegetables

seasoning with salt and pepper

pesto aoli (fresh pesto aoli)

6 tbsp. green pesto (fresh, pre-made)

fresh mayonnaise, 200 g (7 oz)

2 smashed garlic cloves

To make the pesto aoli, combine all of the ingredients in a mixing bowl. Remove from the equation.

In a medium mixing bowl, combine the breadcrumbs, lemon zest, a pinch of chili flakes, a sprinkling of thyme, and some seasoning. In a separate bowl, whisk together the flour and the eggs.

Using kitchen paper, pat the mozzarella balls dry. The balls should be floured first, then dipped in the egg, and last rolled in the breadcrumb mixture. To make a double layer, repeat the process with the egg and breadcrumbs.

Vegetable oil should be half-filled in a saucepan or deep-fat fryer. Heat to 180°C (350°F) just before serving, or until a cube of bread sizzles and turns brown in 10–15 seconds. Lower batches of crumbed mozzarella into the hot oil with a spider strainer or slotted spoon and fry for 3–4 minutes, until golden brown. Remove the pan from the heat and drain on kitchen paper.

Serve with a fresh pesto aoli right away.

To make the tomato, bocconcini, and basil tricolore salad, slice four tomatoes and combine them with a small handful of basil leaves and 300 g (10 oz) bocconcini in a large salad bowl. Drizzle 4 tablespoons extra virgin olive oil over the top and squeeze the juice of 1 lemon over the top. Serve with ciabatta bread and seasonings. Cooking time is 10 minutes total.

Chapter Ten

FLORENTINE EGGS

4 servings

10 minutes total cooking time

15 g (12 oz) butter, with a little extra to butter the muffins

spinach leaves, 200 g (7 oz)

4 muffins, half-sized

4 quail eggs

3 tblsp. parsley, chopped

ready-made hollandaise sauce, 200 mL (7 fl oz)

seasoning with salt and pepper

Bring a small pot half-filled with water to a boil. Meanwhile, in a large saucepan, melt the butter, add the spinach, and simmer, stirring constantly, for 1–2 minutes, until wilted. Salt & pepper to taste.

Cut-side up, toast the muffins under a preheated medium grill until lightly browned. Meanwhile, poach the eggs in boiling water for 1–2 minutes, until the whites are firm and the yolks are soft, 2 at a time.

Warm the muffins, butter them, then split the spinach among them and top with an egg. Pour the hollandaise over the eggs and stir in the parsley. Serve immediately with freshly ground black pepper on top.

Melt 25 g (1 oz) butter in a pot and cook 2 finely sliced leeks over medium heat, stirring, for 3–4 minutes, until tender and beginning to brown, for eggs florentine with leek & cheese sauce. Remove from the heat and stir in 25 g (1 oz) plain flour, then add 400 ml (14 fl oz) milk a bit at a time, blending well between additions. Return to the fire and bring to a boil, stirring frequently, until thickened, adding 1 teaspoon prepared english mustard. 2 tablespoons parmesan cheese, freshly grated Cook and prepare the spinach, eggs, and muffins as directed for eggs florentine, but use the leek and cheese sauce instead of the parsley hollandaise, and top with more grated parmesan if desired. Cooking time is 20 minutes total.

Chapter Eleven

ROSTIS

Rostis of spring onions with a spicy sauce

4 servings

30 minutes total cooking time

cooked potatoes, 875 g (134 pound) (king edward or maris piper)

6 finely chopped spring onions

2 garlic cloves, cut very coarsely

1 lightly beaten big egg

4 tbsp sunflower seed oil

To serve, lime wedges

Salsa

2 plum tomatoes, deseeded and cut roughly

1 deseeded and finely chopped red chili

1 halved and thinly sliced tiny red onion

4 tablespoons fresh coriander, freshly chopped

2 peeled, stoned, and coarsely cut avocados

2 limes' juice

1 tbsp avocado butter

seasoning with salt and pepper

To make the salsa, combine all of the ingredients in a mixing dish. Season generously with salt and pepper and keep aside until ready to serve.

Potatoes should be peeled and coarsely grated. Mix in the spring onions, garlic, and egg with your fingertips until everything is evenly combined.

Half of the oil should be heated in a large nonstick frying pan over high heat.

Divide the potato mixture into 8 parts in stages. 4 of the parts should be spooned into the oil and patted down to make a rostis measuring 8–10 cm (3–4 in) in diameter. Cook for 3–4 minutes on each side, then transfer to a large nonstick baking sheet with care. To make 8 rostis, repeat with the remaining oil and potato mixture.

Serve the rostis with the salsa and lime wedges on the side.

12 sliced spring onions, 400 g (13 oz) cooked, cubed potatoes, 2 crushed garlic cloves, 4 teaspoons chopped fresh coriander leaves, 600 ml (1 pint) hot vegetable stock, and 500 ml (17 fl oz) milk in a saucepan for spring onion & potato broth Bring to a boil, then reduce to a low heat for 5–6 minutes, or until blistering hot. Season to taste and serve right away. Cooking time is 10 minutes total.

Chapter Twelve

BOATS

Boats made of walnuts, gorgonzola, and pears

4 servings

10 minutes total cooking time

1 cored and finely sliced ripe pear

2 tablespoons sour cream

65 g (212 oz) crumbled gorgonzola cheese

20 Belgian chicory leaves, red or green (or a mixture of both)

25 g (1 oz) roasted walnuts, roughly chopped

Sprinkle with olive oil

In a small bowl, combine the pear, crème fraîche, and gorgonzola.

Arrange the chicory leaves on a serving tray and pour a small amount of the pear mixture onto each leaf's base.

Serve with a drizzle of olive oil and a sprinkle of chopped nuts on top of the filling.

Trim any coarse or bruised outer leaves from 8 large heads red chicory for baked chicory with gorgonzola. Place them in a baking dish that will fit them tightly in a single layer. Season with 6 tablespoons olive oil and salt and pepper to taste. Sprinkle 100 g (312 oz) crumbled gorgonzola cheese and 1 lemon juice on top. Cook for 20 minutes at 180°C (350°F), gas mark 4 in a preheated oven. Serve with the liquids from the baking dish and 4 tablespoons chopped toasted walnuts on top before serving. Cooking time is 30 minutes total.

Chapter Thirteen

BRUSCHETTA

Bruschetta with Borlotti beans and peppers

4 servings

Cooking time total: 20 minutes

8 pieces from 1 large baguette

3 tablespoons extra virgin olive oil

1 clove of garlic

Borlotti beans, rinsed and drained, 400 g (13 oz)

3 sliced spring onions

100 g (312 oz) jarred roasted red peppers, drained and thinly sliced

6 finely shredded basil leaves

seasoning with salt and pepper

Drizzle 2 tablespoons olive oil over the baguette pieces and place on a baking sheet. Cook for 2–3 minutes on each side on a preheated hot grill, until browned and golden.

Garlic cloves should be rubbed on each slice of bread.

In a bowl, lightly crush the drained borlotti beans and spring onions together with a fork.

Add the red pepper, basil, the remaining olive oil, and a pinch of salt and pepper to taste.

Serve right away by spooning the bean mixture onto the toasted baguette slices.

To make a quick bean salad, combine a 400 g (13 oz) can rinsed and drained borlotti beans, 3 sliced spring onions, 100 g (312 oz) drained and chopped roasted red peppers from a jar, 3 chopped tomatoes, 4–5 shredded basil leaves, 2 tablespoons olive oil, and 1 tablespoon balsamic vinegar in a large serving bowl. Cooking time is 10 minutes total.

Chapter Fourteen

PITAS

Pitas with a red pepper dip and herbs

4 servings

Cooking time total: 20 minutes

5 tablespoons extra virgin olive oil

1 finely chopped shallot

Walnut halves, 100 g (312 oz)

200 g (7 oz) jarred ready-roasted red peppers

1 smashed garlic clove

1 teaspoon cumin powder

pomegranate molasses, 1 tablespoon

a total of four pita breads

a handful of parsley, chopped

a pinch of mint, chopped

kosher salt (coarse)

In a frying pan, heat 1 tablespoon of the oil, then add the shallot and cook for 3 minutes, or until softened. Allow to cool.

In a dry frying pan, toast the walnut halves for 3 minutes, until lightly browned, then set aside to cool. Combine the walnuts, shallot, peppers, garlic, cumin, pomegranate molasses, and 2 tablespoons of the oil in a blender and blend until smooth. Season with salt and pepper to taste.

In the meantime, cut the pitas in half horizontally and into wedges. Brush the remaining oil over the wedges, along with the herbs. Place on a baking sheet, sprinkle with coarse sea salt, and bake for 5–7 minutes, or until golden and crisp, in a preheated oven at 190°C (375°F), gas mark 5. Serve with the red pepper dip on the side.

Lightly toast 25 g (1 oz) walnut halves in a dry frying pan for the herb and roasted pepper salad. 1 tablespoon sherry vinegar and 3 tablespoons olive oil, whisked together Toss with 150 g (5 oz) mixed herb salad and 2 strips of ready-roasted red peppers. Season with salt and pepper to taste. Arrange on a platter, then top with walnuts and crumbled soft goats' cheese (50 g/2 oz). Cooking time is 10 minutes total.

Chapter Fifteen

BAKED BRIE

Brie baked with maple syrup

4 servings

Cooking time total: 20 minutes

Whole baby brie or camembert, 300 g (10 oz)

pecans, 25 g (1 oz)

maple syrup (three tablespoons)

3 tbsp. dark brown sugar, soft

sprigs of thyme

To serve, crusty bread

Return the cheese to its wooden box after removing any plastic packaging. Place on a baking sheet and bake for 15 minutes at 200°C (400°F), gas mark 6 in a preheated oven.

In a small frying pan, toast the pecans for 3–5 minutes, until lightly toasted, then set aside. Bring the maple syrup and sugar to a boil in a small saucepan. Cook for 1 minute, or until the mixture becomes frothy.

Remove the cheese from the oven and score it in the center with a small cross. Drizzle the maple syrup on top, scatter the pecans and thyme on top, and serve with crusty bread.

1 tablespoon maple syrup, 1 teaspoon mustard, 1 tablespoon white wine vinegar, and 3 tablespoons olive oil are combined in a brie salad with maple dressing. Season with salt and pepper, then toss with 200 g (7 oz) mixed salad leaves. Serve with 25 g (1 oz) roasted pecans on the side. 125 g (4 oz) brie should be cut into thick pieces. Place the brie on a baking sheet and heat for 1 minute or until it begins to melt under a hot grill. To serve, scatter the toppings over the salad. Cooking time is 10 minutes total.

Chapter Sixteen

CROSTINI

crostini with broad beans and peas

(serves 6)

Cooking time total: 20 minutes

olive oil, 75 ml (3 fl oz)

a single lemon

2 peeled garlic cloves

wide beans, 300 g (10 oz)

Peas, 300 g (10 oz)

Mint leaves, a handful

6 sourdough bread slices

seasoning with salt and pepper

to assist

2 finely sliced radishes

a smidgeon of pea shoots

flakes of pecorino cheese

In a small pan, combine the oil, 3 strips of lemon rind, and the garlic cloves and simmer for 7–10 minutes over very low heat. Remove the lemon rind from the pan and set it aside.

In a pan of lightly salted boiling water, cook the wide beans and peas for 3 minutes, or until just tender. To cool, drain and rinse under cold running water. Remove the broad beans from their shells and peel them.

Place the majority of the peas and beans in a blender, along with the mint and cooked garlic, and pulse to form a rough purée. Season to taste.

Toast the bread slices, then cut them in half and put them on a serving tray. Spread the purée over top and top with the peas and wide beans you saved. Serve garnished with radishes, pea shoots, and pecorino cheese shavings.

Cook 100 g (312 oz) each of peas and wide beans in lightly salted boiling water for 3 minutes until mushy, drain, and cool under cold running water for pea & broad bean salad. Toss 150 g (5 oz) salad leaves with 3 tablespoons olive oil and 1 tablespoon lemon juice, seasoning to taste. To serve, arrange the peas and beans on serving dishes and sprinkle with pecorino cheese shavings. Cooking time is 10 minutes total.

Chapter Seventeen

POACHED EGGS

with asparagus

4 servings

10 minute total cooking time

Asparagus spears, 700 g (1 lb 6 oz)

1 tablespoon extra virgin olive oil

4 quail eggs

Parmesan cheese, 40 g (134 oz)

Remove and discard the woody ends of the asparagus spears. Sprinkle the oil into a griddle pan that has been heated to high temperatures.

Meanwhile, boil some water in a frying pan for the eggs.

Place the asparagus on the griddle and cook, rotating occasionally, until the ends are slightly browned.

Stir the boiling water rapidly, then drop the cracked eggs into the center one at a time — the swirling water will help the egg white collect around the yolk and keep the egg's shape. 4–5 minutes in the oven, then remove with a slotted spoon.

Serve the asparagus with the poached eggs on four hot plates.

Make curly parmesan shavings with a vegetable peeler and place on top of the asparagus.

In a frying pan, heat 1 tablespoon oil, then add 6 chopped asparagus spears, 2 sliced spring onions, and 3–4 sliced chestnut mushrooms, cooking for 5–6 minutes. To ensure that all of the eggs cook, whisk together 5 eggs and 4 tablespoons milk and pour into the pan, tilting the pan and stirring the egg with a spatula as needed. Place under a prepared high grill for 1–2 minutes, until brown, then top with 25 g (1 oz) grated parmesan. Serve with a green salad and fresh potatoes, cut into quarters. Cooking time is 20 minutes total.

Chapter Eighteen

OMELETTE

with chickpeas and spinach

4 servings

Cooking time total: 20 minutes

2 tablespoons extra virgin olive oil

1 big chopped onion

1 red pepper, de-seeded, cored, and sliced

12 teaspoon smoked paprika (hot or sweet)

chickpeas, 400 g (13 oz) can, drained and rinsed

100 g (312 oz) washed and roughly cut spinach leaves

5 gently beaten eggs

green olives, pitted and roughly chopped, 75 g (3 oz)

150 g (5 oz) grated cheddar cheese

seasoning with salt and pepper

In a large nonstick frying pan, heat the olive oil. Cook for 7–8 minutes, until the onion and pepper are tender and golden. Cook for 1 minute, stirring often, after adding the paprika and chickpeas. Cook until the spinach leaves are slightly wilted.

Stir the beaten eggs into the pan to mix them. Cook for 4–5 minutes, without stirring, until almost set.

Add the olives and shredded cheddar and place under a hot grill, keeping the handle away from the flames. 4–5 minutes on the grill, or until golden and set. Serve immediately after slicing into wedges.

In a large frying pan, heat 2 tablespoons olive oil for chickpea and spinach salad with poached eggs. Cook for 7–8 minutes with 1 sliced onion and 1 deseeded and sliced red pepper. Cook for 1 minute, stirring regularly, after adding 12 teaspoon hot smoked or sweet paprika and 400 g (13 oz) can chickpeas, drained and rinsed. Poach 4 eggs in a large pan of gently simmering water in the meantime. Toss the chickpea mixture with 200 g (7 oz) baby spinach leaves for a quick toss, then divide among 4 serving plates. Serve immediately with a poached egg on top of each salad. Cooking time is 10 minutes total.

Chapter Nineteen

BEAN BURGERS

topped with a garlicky yogurt sauce

4 servings

30 minutes total cooking time

3 tablespoons oil (vegetable)

1 finely chopped onion

1 sliced garlic clove

400 g (13 oz) drained and rinsed kidney beans

400 g (13 oz) drained and rinsed black-eyed beans

1 tablespoon pureed tomatoes

paprika, 1 teaspoon (optional)

4 tablespoons flat leaf parsley, finely chopped

1 lightly beaten tiny egg

fresh white breadcrumbs, 100 g (312 oz)

Natural yogurt, 250 mL (8 fl oz)

1 smashed tiny garlic clove

lemon juice, 2 tablespoons

seasoning with salt and pepper

4 warmed soft flour tortillas to serve

Garnish with lettuce leaves

In a small frying pan, heat 2 tablespoons of the oil and gently sauté the onion for 6–7 minutes. Cook for another 2–3 minutes, or until the garlic is really tender and brown.

Meanwhile, combine both cans of beans, tomato purée, paprika, and half of the parsley in the large bowl of a food processor. Pulse the contents until it forms a coarse paste. Add the egg, breadcrumbs, and sautéed onion mixture to a mixing bowl. Season with salt and pepper, then thoroughly combine and form into four large burgers.

In a large nonstick frying pan, heat the remaining oil and gently cook the burgers for 8–10 minutes, flipping once, until crisp and brown.

Meanwhile, combine the yogurt, crushed garlic, remaining parsley, and lemon juice in a mixing bowl. Set aside after seasoning with salt and pepper.

Serve the burgers with warmed tortillas and yogurt, with lettuce leaves on the side.

To make mixed bean hummus, combine a 400 g (13 oz) can rinsed and drained mixed beans, 1 tablespoon tomato purée, 1 teaspoon paprika, 4 tablespoons finely chopped flat leaf parsley, 1 tiny crushed garlic clove, and 2 teaspoons lemon juice in a food processor and puree until smooth. Season to taste with salt and pepper, then serve with a variety of raw veggies for dipping. Cooking time is 10 minutes total.

Chapter Twenty

FILLED PEPPERS

filled with feta

4 servings

Cooking time total: 20 minutes

1 tablespoon extra virgin olive oil

4 peppers, long

2 beaten egg yolks

200 g (8 oz) crumbled feta cheese

natural yogurt, 3 tablespoons

12 lemon rind, finely grated

1 teaspoon oregano, chopped

Rub the peppers with the oil, place them in a grill pan, and cook for 5 minutes, rotating once, until they are just soft. Allow it cool for a few minutes before cutting in half lengthwise and removing the seeds.

In a food processor, combine the egg yolks, three-quarters of the feta, the yogurt, and the lemon rind until smooth. Fill the peppers halfway with the mixture, then top with the remaining feta crumbles and oregano.

Return to the grill and cook for another 5–7 minutes, or until golden and fully done. Allow it cool for a few minutes before serving.

4 large sheets of foil, lightly greased for spicy baked feta with peppers Top each sheet with 1 thinly sliced red onion, 2 chopped ready-roasted peppers, and a handful of halved cherry tomatoes. Place a 100 g (312 oz) feta cheese chunk on top of each serving, along with a handful of chopped oregano and 1 sliced red chili. Drizzle a little olive oil on top, then fold the foil in half to create sealed packets. Place on a baking sheet and bake for 20 minutes at 200°C (400°F), gas mark 6 in a preheated oven. With plenty of crusty bread, of course. Cooking time is 30 minutes total.

Chapter Twenty-one

CIABATTA TOAST WITH VEGETABLES

4 servings

10 minutes total cooking time

5 tbsp olive oil, plus a little extra for drizzling

12 aubergine, thinly sliced and trimmed

1 loaf of ciabatta

4 tablespoons pesto verde

1 finely sliced big beef tomato

4 mozzarella cheese slices

Pepper

In a large, heavy-bottomed frying pan, heat the oil and cook the aubergine slices in batches for 1–2 minutes on each side, until browned and tender. Keep warm by removing with a fish slice.

In the meantime, cut the ciabatta bread in half lengthwise, then in half again widthwise. Place cut-side up on the grill rack and cook for 1 minute on a preheated high grill until brown.

1 tablespoon pesto should be spread on each ciabatta toastie. Top with heated aubergine slices, tomato slices, and mozzarella slices, in that order. Drizzle 1 tablespoon olive oil over each toastie, then return to the grill for another 2 minutes, or until the mozzarella is melted and beginning to color in spots.

Season with pepper and serve while still hot.

In a large frying pan, gently heat 4 tablespoons olive oil and sauté 1 sliced aubergine in batches over high heat for 1–2 minutes on each side until browned and soft, for mediterranean vegetable gratin. Layer 3 sliced large beef tomatoes, 2 x 150 g (5 oz) packs mozzarella cheese, drained and thinly sliced, and 6 tablespoons green pesto in a large, shallow gratin dish, seasoning between layers. Cook for 8–10 minutes, until brown and bubbling, under a preheated high grill with 3 tablespoons freshly grated parmesan cheese. Cooking time is 30 minutes total.

Chapter Twenty-two

SOUP 1

with lettuce, peas, and tarragon

4 servings

Cooking time total: 20 minutes

2 tablespoons unsalted butter

8 trimmed and sliced spring onions

frozen peas, 750 g (112 lb)

1 tablespoon tarragon leaves, chopped

1 finely shredded romaine lettuce

1 litre hot vegetable stock (134 pints)

double cream, 2 tablespoons

seasoning with salt and pepper

Garnish with sprigs of tarragon (optional)

In a large saucepan over medium heat, melt the butter. Cook, stirring constantly, for 2 minutes after adding the spring onions.

Combine the peas, half of the tarragon, and the lettuce in a mixing bowl. 1 minute of cooking

Bring the stock to a boil, then reduce to a low heat and cook for 5 minutes, or until the vegetables are soft.

Pour the soup into a blender and blend until smooth, adding the remaining tarragon if needed. Season with salt and pepper to taste.

Divide the soup among four bowls, stir in the cream, and season with black pepper. If desired, garnish with tarragon sprigs.

Separate the leaves of 2 washed romaine lettuces and set them in a large, wide salad bowl with 8 sliced spring onions, 4 sliced plum tomatoes, 500 g (1 lb) blanched peas, and 12 sliced radishes for a lettuce, pea, tomato, and spring onion salad. To make the dressing, combine 1 lemon's juice, 6 tablespoons olive oil, 1 teaspoon dijon mustard, 2 tablespoons finely chopped tarragon, and 2 teaspoons clear honey in a mixing bowl. Season with salt and pepper, then pour over the salad components. Toss well to combine and serve. Cooking time is 10 minutes total.

Chapter Twenty-three

SOUP 2

with roasted tomatoes

4 servings

30 minutes total cooking time

1 kilo (2 lb) ripe tomatoes, peeled and halved

4 unpeeled garlic cloves

2 tablespoons extra virgin olive oil

1 chopped onion

1 sliced carrot

1 sliced celery stick

1 cored, deseeded, and chopped red pepper

700 mL (1 pint 3 oz) vegetable stock, hot

seasoning with salt and pepper

4 tbsp. grated parmesan cheese (to serve)

In a roasting pan, combine the tomato halves and garlic cloves. Roast for 20 minutes at 200°C (400°F), gas mark 6 in a preheated oven with 1 tablespoon of olive oil and some pepper.

After 10 minutes, in a saucepan, heat the remaining olive oil and sauté the onion, carrot, celery, and red pepper for 10 minutes over low heat.

Remove the garlic cloves from their shells and squeeze the garlic flesh into the pan with the sautéed vegetables after the tomatoes are done.

Along with the stock, add the roast tomatoes and all of their juices. Blend the soup until smooth with a hand blender, a food processor, or a blender. Season with salt and pepper to taste.

If required, reheat, then serve with grated parmesan cheese on top.

In a skillet, heat 2 tablespoons olive oil and sauté 1 chopped onion, 1 chopped carrot, 1 chopped celery stick, and 700 g (1112 lb) chopped tomatoes for 5 minutes to make a quick tomato soup. Add a 400 g (13 oz) diced tomato can and 900 ml (112 quarts) boiling vegetable stock to the pot. Remove from the heat after 10 minutes and stir in a small handful of basil leaves. Blend the soup until smooth with a hand blender, a food processor, or a blender. Season to taste and drizzle with extra virgin olive oil before serving. Cooking time is 20 minutes total.

Chapter Twenty-four

SOUP 3

with egg and greens from the Far East

4 servings

30 minutes total cooking time

4 green onions

pak choi, coarsely chopped, 100 g (312 oz)

2 tablespoons oil (vegetable)

fresh root ginger, finely grated, 2.5 cm (1 in)

2 finely chopped garlic cloves

jasmine rice, 200 g (7 oz)

Rice wine, 100 ml (312 fl oz)

2 tblsp soy sauce (optional)

1 teaspoon vinegar (rice wine)

1 litre hot vegetable stock (134 pints)

4 quail eggs

1 tbsp. chili oil (for drizzling)

Spring onions should be finely sliced, with the white and green sections kept separate. In a bowl, combine the green parts with the pak choi and leave aside.

In a saucepan, gradually heat the oil. Stir-fry the onion whites, ginger, and garlic for 2–3 minutes once the pan is heated.

Stir in the rice, then add the wine and allow to bubble for about a minute.

Stir in the soy sauce, vinegar, and stock and cook for 10–12 minutes, stirring regularly. Cook for another 2–3 minutes after adding the saved spring onions and pak choi. Poach the eggs in two batches in the meantime.

To serve, spoon the soup into four shallow soup bowls, top with a poached egg, and drizzle with chili oil.

Place 300 g (10 oz) blanched and roughly chopped pak choi, 6 sliced spring onions, and 500 g (1 lb) cooked jasmine rice in a salad dish for oriental rice & asian green salad. 1 crushed garlic clove, 1 teaspoon grated ginger, 14 teaspoon chilli oil, 2 teaspoons light soy sauce, the juice of 2 limes, a dash of rice wine vinegar, and 4 tablespoons vegetable oil combine to make a dressing. Season with salt and pepper, then pour over the salad and toss well to combine before serving. Cooking time is 10 minutes total.

Chapter Twenty-five

SOUP 4

with sweet potatoes and red peppers

4 servings

Cooking time total: 20 minutes

2 tablespoons oil (vegetable)

1 chopped red onion

1 cored, deseeded, and chopped red pepper

550 g (1 lb 2 oz) peeled and sliced sweet potatoes

14 teaspoon cumin powder

a total of 8 cherry tomatoes

vegetable stock, 1.2 litres (2 pints)

25 g (1 oz) chopped creamed coconut

seasoning with salt and pepper

to assist

Yogurt made from natural ingredients

sprigs of fresh coriander

In a medium saucepan, heat the oil, then add the onion and pepper and sauté for 3–4 minutes. Cook for another 2–3 minutes after adding the sweet potatoes, cumin, and tomatoes.

Pour in the stock, bring to a boil, and then reduce to a low heat for 12 minutes. Cook for another 2–3 minutes after adding the creamed coconut. Blend the soup until smooth using a hand-held blender or food processor.

Serve with a dollop of natural yogurt and a sprig of coriander, seasoning with salt and pepper.

Slice 900 g (134 pound) sweet potatoes into wedges for a warm sweet potato wedges salad. 2 crushed garlic cloves, 4 tablespoons olive oil, 2 teaspoons minced sage, 1 teaspoon paprika, and some salt and pepper in a large mixing bowl Toss the potato with the herb and spice mixture, then place it in a roasting tin and roast for 25 minutes at 200°C (400°F), gas mark 6. Toss potato wedges with 250 g (8 oz) baby spinach leaves and 4 sliced spring onions before serving. Cooking time is 30 minutes total.

Chapter Twenty-six

SOUP 5

with lentils, mustard, and chickpeas

4 servings

Cooking time total: 20 minutes

12 tblsp. coconut or olive oil

a quarter teaspoon of mustard seeds

12 teaspoon cumin powder

12 teaspoon turmeric powder

1 small sliced onion

a 1.5-cm (34-inch) piece of freshly cut fresh root ginger

1 finely sliced garlic clove

Red split lentils, 100 g (312 oz)

250 g (8 oz) washed and drained canned chickpeas

heated vegetable stock, 900 mL (112 quarts)

infant spinach leaves, 50 g (2 oz)

seasoning with salt and pepper

In a saucepan, heat the oil and add the dry spices. Add the onion, ginger, and garlic when the mustard seeds begin to pop, and simmer until the onion softens.

Stir in the lentils and chickpeas until fully combined. Bring the stock to a boil, then reduce to a low heat and cook for 14–16 minutes, or until the lentils are tender.

Season to taste after stirring in the spinach until it has wilted. To serve, ladle the soup into bowls.

In a large frying pan, heat 3 tablespoons olive oil, add 1 deseeded and chopped red chili, 12 teaspoon mustard seeds, 2 sliced garlic cloves, and a 2.5-cm (1-inch) piece of peeled and grated root ginger, and sauté for 2 minutes. Remove from the heat and add 1 small sliced red onion, a 400 g (13 oz) can of rinsed and drained lentils and chickpeas, the juice of 12 lemon, and 2 tablespoons chopped sun-dried tomatoes. Stir together, then toss with 60 g (214 oz) rocket leaves and 150 g (5 oz) crumbled feta cheese in a serving bowl. Cooking time is 10 minutes total.

Chapter Twenty-seven

GREEN GAZPACHO

with ice

4 servings

20-minute total preparation time

a couple of celery sticks (including leaves)

1 deseeded little green pepper

1 big peeled cucumber

3 stale white bread slices (crusts removed)

1 deseeded fresh green chili

4 cloves of garlic

1 teaspoon honey, transparent

150 g (5 oz) gently toasted walnuts

Baby spinach, 200 g (7 oz)

basil leaves, 50 g (2 oz)

4 tbsp apple cider vinegar

250 mL (8 oz) extra virgin olive oil, with a little more for drizzling

6 tablespoons plain yogurt

16 fl oz (475 ml) iced water

a few cubes of ice

seasoning with salt and pepper

To serve, ready-made croutons

Chop the celery, pepper, cucumber, bread, chili, and garlic into small pieces.

Add the honey, walnuts, spinach, basil, vinegar, oil, yogurt, most of the iced water, and ice cubes to a blender and blend until smooth. Season to taste. Blend the soup until it is completely smooth. If necessary, add more chilled water to get the desired consistency.

If required, season the soup with salt and pepper.

Serve in cold dishes with croutons and olive oil drizzled on top.

4 thinly sliced celery sticks, 1 sliced cucumber, 1 deseeded and thinly sliced green pepper, and 100 g (312 oz) baby spinach go into a large wide bowl for a green vegetable salad. In a bowl, whisk together 150 mL (1/4 pint) natural yogurt, 1 crushed garlic clove, 1 teaspoon clear honey, and 1 finely diced green chili to make a dressing. Before serving, drizzle over the salad

and top with a tiny handful of ready-made croutons. Cooking time is 10 minutes total.

Chapter Twenty-eight

SPICY LENTILS SOUP

4 servings

30 minutes total cooking time

2 tbsp sunflower seed oil

1 finely sliced garlic clove

1 teaspoon fresh root ginger, grated

1 finely chopped red chili

1 finely chopped onion

1 tablespoon sweet smoked paprika, with a little extra to sprinkle on top

700 g (112 lb) peeled and finely cut carrots

150 g (5 oz) rinsed and drained red split lentils

Single cream, 150 mL (14 pint)

1 litre hot vegetable stock (134 pints)

crème fraîche, 100 mL (312 fl oz)

a small handful of fresh coriander leaves, chopped

seasoning with salt and pepper

Onions that have been caramelized

1 tablespoon unsalted butter

1 tablespoon extra virgin olive oil

1 finely sliced onion

In a heavy-bottomed saucepan, heat the sunflower oil, then add the garlic, ginger, red chili, onion, and smoky paprika and cook, stirring, for 1–2 minutes over medium-high heat. Bring the carrots, lentils, cream, and stock to a boil, then decrease the heat to medium and cook for 15–20 minutes, uncovered.

Meanwhile, to create the caramelized onions, melt the butter and olive oil in a frying pan, then add the onion and cook for 12–15 minutes, or until golden brown and caramelized. Keep heated by draining on kitchen paper.

Blend the lentil mixture in the pan with an electric stick blender or food processor until smooth, then season well.

Pour into bowls and top with a dollop of crème fraiche, chopped coriander leaves, and caramelized onions. Before serving, sprinkling with smoked paprika.

2 rinsed and drained 400 g (12 oz) green lentils, 2 peeled and roughly grated carrots, 1 finely chopped red chili, 4 sliced spring onions, and a large handful of chopped fresh coriander leaves go into a salad dish for spicy lentil & carrot salad. 1 teaspoon sweet smoked paprika, 150 mL (1/4 pint) shop-bought fresh french salad dressing Season to taste, stir to combine, and serve. Cooking time is 10 minutes total.

Chapter Twenty-nine

TUSCAN BEAN AND TRUFFLES SOUP

4 servings

Cooking time total: 20 minutes

2 tablespoons extra virgin olive oil

1 chopped onion

2 chopped garlic cloves

400 g (13 oz) rinsed and drained cannellini beans

Butter beans, 400 g (13 ounce) can, rinsed and drained

400 g (13 oz) chopped tomatoes in a can

12 shredded savoy cabbage

12 tbsp rosemary, chopped

Vegetable stock, 850 mL (112 pints)

1 teaspoon oil de truffe

seasoning with salt and pepper

To serve, 25 g (1 oz) grated parmesan cheese

In a medium saucepan, heat the oil, then add the onion and sauté for 1–2 minutes, until softened.

Cook for 1 minute after adding the garlic, cannellini beans, and butter beans to the onions.

Pour in the stock and the truffle oil after adding the tomatoes, cabbage, and rosemary to the pan. Combine all ingredients in a large mixing bowl, season with salt and pepper, and bring to a boil. Cook for 10–12 minutes, or until the cabbage is tender.

To serve, divide the soup among four shallow plates and top with parmesan cheese.

To make the tuscan bean and truffle salad, steam 150 g (5 oz) trimmed green beans for 2–3 minutes, then refresh under cold running water before tossing with a 400 g (13 oz) can each of cannellini and butter beans, rinsed and drained, 125 g (4 oz) halved baby tomatoes, 4 sliced spring onions, and 2 tablespoons chopped parsley. Toss the salad with 3 tablespoons olive oil, 2 teaspoons truffle oil, 1 tablespoon balsamic vinegar, and 1 teaspoon clear honey before serving. Cooking time is 10 minutes total.

Chapter Thirty

GOAT CHEESE AND BEETS SALAD

4 servings

10 minutes total cooking time

2 tablespoons extra virgin olive oil

3 peeled and shredded raw beets

4 tblsp balsamic vinaigrette

sunflower seeds, 2 teaspoons

Goat cheese, 200 g (7 oz)

Rocket leaves, 75 g (3 oz)

2 tbsp olive oil (extra virgin)

Pepper

In a frying pan, heat the olive oil, then add the beetroot and cook for 3–4 minutes. Season with salt and pepper, then add the vinegar and simmer for 30 seconds over high heat.

Meanwhile, dry-fry the sunflower seeds in a nonstick frying pan over medium-low heat for 2 minutes, tossing often, until golden and toasted. Remove from the equation.

Divide the beets among four plates. Crumble the cheese on top, then scatter the rocket on top.

Serve with a drizzle of extra virgin olive oil and roasted sunflower seeds on top.

In a saucepan, heat 1 tablespoon olive oil, add 1 chopped onion, and cook for 2–3 minutes for beetroot soup with goats' cheese. Bring to a boil 3 grated raw beetroot, 600 ml (1 pint) hot vegetable stock, and a 400 g (13 oz) diced tomato can. Reduce the heat to low and continue to cook for another 8–10 minutes, or until the beetroot is soft. Blend the soup until smooth using a hand-held blender or food processor, then season to taste. To serve, ladle into dishes and top with 100 g (312 oz) goats' cheese crumbles. Cooking time is 20 minutes total.

Chapter Thirty-one

PUMPKIN AND APPLES SOUP

4 servings

30 minutes total cooking time

2 tablespoons extra virgin olive oil

1 chopped onion

600 g pumpkin flesh, chopped into chunks (1 lb 5 oz)

1 peeled, cored, and chopped bramley apple

2 peeled and sliced tomatoes

Vegetable stock, 900 mL (112 pints)

Double cream, 100 mL (312 fl oz)

1 tablespoon flat leaf parsley, finely chopped

seasoning with salt and pepper

In a large saucepan, heat the olive oil and sauté the onion for 3–4 minutes.

Stir in the pumpkin to combine it with the onions. Combine the apple and chopped tomatoes in a mixing bowl.

Pour in the stock, bring to a boil, then reduce to a low heat and continue to cook, covered, for 20 minutes, or until the pumpkin is soft.

Allow for some cooling time before adding the cream. Blend the soup until smooth with a hand blender, a food processor, or a blender.

If necessary, reheat gently, season, and serve immediately, garnished with chopped parsley.

Cut 1 kg (2 lb) pumpkin flesh into small dice for the pumpkin and chickpea salad. Roast for 15 minutes at 200°C (400°F), gas mark 6 in a preheated oven with 1 crushed garlic clove, 12 teaspoon of cumin, and 2 tablespoons olive oil. Combine the roasted pumpkin, 400 g (13 oz) rinsed and drained chickpeas, 1 small chopped red onion, 150 g (5 oz) crumbled feta cheese, 50 g (2 oz) sun-dried tomatoes, and 50 g (2 oz) rocket leaves in a mixing bowl. Dress with store-bought Italian salad dressing before serving. Cooking time is 20 minutes total.

Salad with watermelon and haloumi (serves 4) 4

10 minutes total cooking time

Haloumi cheese, 200 g (7 oz), cut into 8 slices

1 lime, finely grated zest and juice

2 thinly chopped spring onions

2 tblsp flat leaf parsley, chopped

2 teaspoons mint, chopped

1 tbsp avocado butter

wild rocket leaves, 150 g (5 oz)

12 oz. peeled, seeded, and chopped watermelon

12 tbsp. coarsely chopped red onion

Green olives filled with almonds, 100 g (312 oz)

pomegranate molasses, 1 tablespoon

to taste 1–2 tablespoons chili paste

Pomegranate seeds, 100 g (312 oz) (about 1 pomegranate)

Pepper

Preheat the grill to high. Place the haloumi on a foil-lined baking dish with the lime zest, spring onions, and 1 tablespoon each of parsley and mint. Drizzle a little avocado oil over the tray and lay it under the grill for 3–4 minutes, flipping once, until hot and brown.

Arrange the rocket leaves on 4 large dishes in the meantime. In a large mixing basin, combine the watermelon, onion, olives, and remaining parsley and mint. Dress the watermelon and place it on top of the rocket.

Toss the lime juice, pomegranate molasses, remaining avocado oil, and chilli paste in a small bowl to taste, then season with black pepper.

2 slices of grilled haloumi on top of each salad, followed by pomegranate seeds. Drizzle with the dressing before serving.

12 watermelon, peeled, deseeded, and diced for watermelon & feta salad. Arrange on serving plates. Over the watermelon, crumble 200 g (7 oz) feta, then spread 2 finely sliced spring onions, 2 tablespoons chopped mint and parsley, and 100 g (312 oz) black olives. Serve with 100 g (312 oz) pomegranate seeds and 1 tablespoon pomegranate molasses poured on top. Cooking time is 10 minutes total.

Chapter Thirty-two

SPICY SOYA AND NOODLES SALAD

4 servings

15-minute total cooking time

dried soba noodles, 250 g (8 oz)

frozen podded soya beans, 250 g (8 oz)

6 thinly sliced diagonally spring onions

sesame seeds, 2 tblsp

1 inch piece of fresh root ginger, 3 centimeter

1 finely chopped red chili

1 tablespoon sesame oil, roasted

mirin (three tablespoons)

3 tblsp soy sauce (mild)

1 teaspoon honey, transparent

Salt

fresh coriander leaves, chopped to serve as a garnish

In a large pot of lightly salted boiling water, cook the noodles and soya beans for 4–5 minutes, or according to the noodle packet directions. Return to the pan and add the spring onions after draining well. Keep warm by covering.

Heat a frying pan over medium heat until heated, then add the sesame seeds and dry-fry until lightly golden. Remove from the pan and leave aside.

In a mixing bowl, peel and grate the root ginger, then add the remaining ingredients and combine thoroughly. Toss the noodle mixture with the dressing to thoroughly combine it.

Serve in warm bowls with sesame seeds and chopped coriander sprinkled on top.

Bring 800 mL (1 pint 8 fl oz) hot vegetable stock, 1 teaspoon peeled and grated fresh root ginger, 1 chopped red chilli, and 6 finely sliced spring onions to a boil in a saucepan, then add 400 g (12 oz) shop-bought ready-cooked soba noodles and 200 g (7 oz) frozen podded soya beans to a boil. Return to a boil, season with salt and pepper, and serve with chopped fresh coriander leaves and a drizzle of sesame oil. Cooking time is 10 minutes total.

Chapter Thirty-three

BULGUR SALAD

4 servings

Cooking time total: 20 minutes

1 14 pint heated vegetable stock (750 mL)

bulgar wheat, 275 g (9 oz)

4 tblsp. extra virgin olive or vegetable oil

1 halved and thinly sliced large red onion

Tomato juice, 100 mL (312 fl oz)

lime juice (two teaspoons)

175 g (6 oz) crumbled firm goat's cheese

3 tablespoons flat leaf parsley, coarsely chopped

seasoning with salt and pepper

In a large saucepan, bring the vegetable stock to a boil, then add the bulgar wheat and cook for 7 minutes. Remove from the heat and put aside for 5–8 minutes, or until the liquid has been absorbed and the grains are soft.

Meanwhile, in a frying pan, heat 2 tablespoons oil and gently sauté the onion for 7–8 minutes, until tender and golden.

Season with salt and pepper and stir in the remaining oil, tomato juice, and lime juice. With a fork, fold the dressing, onion, goats' cheese, and parsley into the bulgar wheat, and serve in 4 small bowls.

To make goats' cheese couscous, combine 250 g (8 oz) couscous, 1 tablespoon olive or vegetable oil, and a large pinch of salt in a mixing dish. Set aside for 5–8 minutes, until the grains are soft and the liquid has been absorbed, after pouring over 300 mL (12 pint) boiling vegetable stock. Meanwhile, season with salt and pepper 3 tablespoons oil, 100 milliliter (312 fl oz) tomato juice, and 2 tablespoons lime juice. Toss the couscous with the goat's cheese and parsley and serve in serving basins. To serve, drizzle with the dressing and top with 3 sliced spring onions. Cooking time is 10 minutes total.

Chapter Thirty-four

QUINOA AND TOMATOES SALAD

4 servings

30 minutes total cooking time

Quinoa, 150 g (5 oz), washed under cold running water

Boiling water, 300 mL (12 pint)

4 deseeded and sliced yellow or red tomatoes

1 large deseeded and finely chopped green pepper

2 thinly chopped spring onions

kalamata olives, pitted and roughly chopped, 100 g (312 oz)

12 cucumbers, cut lengthwise in half, deseeded, and sliced

1 lemon, grated rind and juice

3 tblsp flat leaf parsley, chopped

3 tablespoons mint, chopped

4 sliced tiny red or white chicory

feta cheese, 100 g (312 oz)

2 teaspoons mixed toasted seeds

Alfalfa sprouts in a small handful

seasoning with salt and pepper

To serve, lemon wedges

Pour the measured boiling water over the quinoa in a medium-sized pot. Cover the pan and cook for 12–15 minutes on low heat. When the seed begins to separate from the germ, it is ready. In a fine sieve, drain the quinoa and chill it under cold running water. Drain thoroughly.

Meanwhile, combine the tomatoes, pepper, spring onions, olives, and cucumber in a large mixing bowl, then add the lemon rind, parsley, and mint.

Season with salt, pepper, and lemon juice to taste after mixing the cooled quinoa with the vegetables. Allow 5–10 minutes for the flavors to come together.

Place the chicory on 4 serving dishes, ladle the quinoa salad on top, then crumble the feta on top. Serve with toasted seeds and alfalfa sprouts sprinkled on top.

Heat 250 g (8 oz) ready-to-eat red and white quinoa or ready-to-eat red mixed nutritious grains according to package directions for minted pea quinoa. Toss the quinoa or grains with 3 tablespoons chopped flat leaf parsley and mint, 125 g

(4 oz) thawed frozen peas, and 2 finely sliced spring onions in a large mixing basin. Season to taste with salt, pepper, and lemon juice and crumble over 100 g (312 oz) wensleydale cheese or any crumbly white cheese. Serve with 2 tablespoons toasted mixed seeds sprinkled over top. Cooking time is 10 minutes total.

Chapter Thirty-five

PANZANELLA

4 servings

30 minutes total cooking time

ripe tomatoes, 300 g (10 oz)

ciabatta bread, 125 g (4 oz)

16 pitted black olives

capers, 3 teaspoons

12 thinly sliced red onion

Red and yellow cherry tomatoes, halved, 300 g (10 oz)

6–8 leaves of basil

1 tablespoon vinegar (red wine)

2 tablespoons extra virgin olive oil

In a strainer over a basin, strain the tomatoes. Squash them with the back of a spoon to release all of the juice into the bowl.

Break up the bread and toss it in with the tomato liquid. Allow it sit for 15 minutes before transferring to a serving plate.

Before serving, scatter the remaining ingredients over the wet bread and drizzle with red wine vinegar and olive oil.

Cut 1 ciabatta loaf into cubes for tomato salad with ciabatta croûtons. In a frying pan, heat 2 tablespoons olive oil and cook the bread cubes till golden. Drain on paper towels. Combine the fried bread with 300 g (10 oz) roughly chopped ripe tomatoes, 16 pitted black olives, 12 sliced red onion, 300 g (10 oz) red and yellow cherry tomatoes, 6–8 torn basil leaves, and 60 g (214 oz) baby spinach leaves in a large mixing bowl. To serve, drizzle with 2 tablespoons extra virgin olive oil and 1 tablespoon red wine vinegar. Cooking time is 10 minutes total.

Chapter Thirty-six

CHICKPEAS SALAD

chickpeas, tomatoes, and peppers

4 servings

30 minutes total cooking time

3 large red peppers, de-seeded, cored, and quartered

6 halved plum tomatoes

4 tablespoons extra virgin olive oil

1 teaspoon seeds of cumin

a quarter-cup of lemon juice

12 teaspoon mustard (dijon)

12 teaspoon honey (clear)

chickpeas, 400 g (13 oz) can, drained

10–12 basil leaves, broken into small pieces

Baby spinach leaves, 100 g (312 oz)

seasoning with salt and pepper

Toss the peppers and tomatoes with 1 tablespoon of the oil and the cumin seeds in a roasting pan. Season with salt and pepper before roasting for 20 minutes at 220°C (425°F), gas mark 7.

To prepare the dressing, whisk together the remaining oil, lemon juice, mustard, and honey.

Take the peppers out of the oven and place them in a basin. Toss in the chickpeas, basil, and spinach, then drizzle with the dressing and serve right away.

In a large saucepan over medium heat, heat 1 tablespoon olive oil, add 1 deseeded and chopped red pepper and 1 diced red onion, and cook for 1–2 minutes for chickpea, tomato, and pepper soup. 3 chopped plum tomatoes and a 400 g (13 oz) container of rinsed and drained chickpeas Season well with 900 mL (112 quarts) vegetable stock. Cook for 4–5 minutes on low heat. Blend until smooth in a hand-held blender or food processor, and sprinkle with olive oil before serving. Cooking time is 10 minutes total.

Chapter Thirty-seven

QUINOA RISOTTO

with asparagus and peas

4 servings

Cooking time total: 20 minutes

quinoa, rinsed, 275 g (9 oz)

Vegetable stock, 600 mL (1 pint)

200 g (7 oz) chopped asparagus

frozen peas, 200 g (7 oz)

1 tablespoon mint leaves, chopped

3 tblsp parmesan cheese, grated

Pepper

In a saucepan, bring the quinoa and stock to a boil, then reduce to a low heat and cook for 12–15 minutes, or until the quinoa is cooked, adding the asparagus and peas approximately 2 minutes before the end of the cooking time.

Drain the quinoa and veggies, then add the mint and 2 tablespoons of the cheese to the pan and season with pepper. Mix thoroughly.

Serve with the remaining parmesan cheese on top.

Unroll a 375 g (12 oz) bag ready-rolled puff pastry onto a baking sheet for the asparagus and pea tart. In a mixing bowl, combine 200 g (7 oz) cream cheese and 1 tablespoon dijon mustard, then spread over the puff pastry, leaving a 1.5 cm (34) border around the edge. Trimmed 300 g (10 oz) asparagus and 100 g (312 oz) defrosted peas go on top. Season with pepper and 50 g (2 oz) grated parmesan cheese, then drizzle with 2 tablespoons olive oil. Preheat the oven to 200°C (400°F), gas mark 6, and bake for 20–22 minutes. Serve alongside a fresh green salad. Cooking time is 30 minutes total.

Chapter Thirty-eight

PIE WITH SPINACH

crispy spinach and feta

4 servings

30 minutes total cooking time

Frozen leaf spinach, 250 g (8 oz)

2 chopped spring onions

1 smashed garlic clove

200 g (7 oz) crumbled feta cheese

2 beaten eggs

a pinch of nutmeg, grated

25 g (1 oz) melted butter

3 tablespoons extra virgin olive oil

5 filo pastry sheets, large

seasoning with salt and pepper

Place the spinach in a colander and thaw it in hot water from the kettle. Squeeze off any excess liquid before mixing in the spring onions, garlic, feta, and eggs. Season with nutmeg and salt & pepper to taste.

Brush the sides and base of a 20 cm (8 inch) springform cake tin with a mixture of butter and oil. Remove the filo pastry from the package and wrap it in moist kitchen paper until ready to use.

Brush 1 sheet of puff pastry with the butter mixture and lay in the tin, allowing the extra pastry to hang over the sides. Brush a second sheet with the butter mixture, turn the tin a little, and position it in the same manner as the first. Continue until the tin's bottom and sides are fully covered.

Fill the tin halfway with the filling, then fold the pastry edges over to cover it, scrunching them up as you go. Brush the top of the pie with a little more butter mixture and bake for 20–25 minutes, until golden and crisp, at 200°C (400°F), gas mark 6.

1 tablespoon lemon juice, 3 tablespoons olive oil, and a teaspoon of ground cumin go into the spinach, feta, and chickpea salad. Season thoroughly with a 400 g (13 oz) can rinsed and drained chickpeas and 12 thinly sliced red onion. Arrange on a serving platter with 125 g (4 oz) baby spinach leaves and 1 chopped ready-roasted red pepper. Serve with 75 g (3 oz) feta cheese crumbled on top. Cooking time is 10 minutes total.

Chapter Thirty-nine

PILAU

Cauliflower pilau with a quick seasoning

4 servings

10 minutes total cooking time

1 oz. raisins, 25 g

tiny cauliflower florets, 400 g (13 oz)

2 tablespoons oil (vegetable)

2 smashed garlic cloves

2 finely sliced spring onions

12 tablespoons curry paste (medium-hot)

500 g (1 lb) steamed pilau rice, ready to eat

fresh coriander leaves, chopped to serve as a garnish

To serve, flatbreads (optional)

Pour 2 tablespoons boiling water over the raisins in a heatproof basin and let aside to soak.

In a large pot of boiling water, cook the cauliflower florets for 4–5 minutes, or until just tender.

Meanwhile, heat the oil in a large skillet and soften the garlic and spring onions for 1 minute over medium heat. To cook the spices, add the curry paste and stir for 1 minute. Cover and cook for 2–3 minutes over medium-low heat with the steamed rice, raisins, and their water.

Drain and fold the cauliflower into the rice. Spoon onto serving dishes, top with coriander, and serve with flatbreads, if desired.

Heat 2 tablespoons vegetable oil in a pan and sauté 1 chopped onion, 2 chopped garlic cloves, and 1 teaspoon cumin seeds over medium heat for 6–7 minutes, stirring occasionally, until softened, for aromatic spiced cauliflower stew. Stir in 2 tablespoons of medium-hot curry paste for 1 minute. Stir in 625 g (1 14 pound) cauliflower florets and a 400 g (13 ounce) rinsed and drained can of chickpeas. Season with salt and pepper, then add a 400 g (13 oz) can cherry or plum tomatoes and 200 ml (7 fl oz) water, cover loosely, and cook for 15–18 minutes, until soft. Serve with a dollop of natural yogurt and chopped fresh coriander leaves. Cooking time is 30 minutes total.

Chapter Forty

EGGS WITH A RANCH FLAVOR

4 servings

30 minutes total cooking time

2 tablespoons extra virgin olive oil

1 thinly sliced onion

1 deseeded and finely chopped red chili

1 smashed garlic clove

1 teaspoon cumin powder

1 teaspoon oregano, dry

cherry tomatoes, 400 g (13 oz)

200 g (7 oz) jarred roasted red and yellow peppers, drained and coarsely chopped

4 quail eggs

seasoning with salt and pepper

4 tablespoons fresh coriander, freshly chopped, to serve as a garnish

In a large frying pan, heat the oil and add the onion, chili, garlic, cumin, and oregano.

Simmer for 5 minutes on low heat, or until soft, then add the tomatoes and peppers and cook for another 5 minutes. If the sauce appears to be dry, a splash of water can be added. Season to taste.

Make four hollows in the mixture and crack an egg into each one before covering the pan. Cook for 5 minutes, or until the eggs are slightly firm to the touch.

Serve immediately with chopped coriander on top.

In a large frying pan, heat 1 tablespoon each olive oil and butter for spicy Mexican-style scrambled eggs. 8 eggs, 1 crushed garlic clove, 1 finely chopped red chili, 1 teaspoon dried oregano, and 1 teaspoon ground cumin, whisked together Season with salt and pepper, then pour into the frying pan and cook, stirring frequently, until the eggs are scrambled and cooked to your desire. Serve with warm tortillas and fresh coriander chopped on top. Cooking time is 10 minutes total.

Chapter Forty-one

POTATO GNOCCHI

4 servings

30 minutes total cooking time

800 g (134 lb) peeled and sliced floury potatoes

1 beaten egg yolk

ordinary flour, 150 g (5 oz)

basil leaves, finely shredded, 15 g (12 oz)

50 g (2 oz) grated parmesan cheese

4 tbsp extra-virgin extra-virgin olive oil

seasoning with salt and pepper

In a saucepan of boiling water, cook the potatoes for 12–15 minutes, or until tender. Drain and mash the potatoes, or use a potato ricer for a silky smooth texture. Bring a separate saucepan of water to a boil.

In a mixing basin, combine the mashed potatoes, egg yolk, flour, and basil. To blend, whisk everything together thoroughly.

Take a teaspoon of the mixture and roll it into a walnut-sized ball in your hand. To make gnocchi, use the prongs of a fork to press the dough into a gnocchi shape. Rep with the rest of the mixture.

Cooking the gnocchi in a saucepan of boiling water should only take 1–2 minutes, and the gnocchi should float when done.

Toss the hot gnocchi with the grated parmesan and a drizzle of olive oil before serving.

In a frying pan, heat 1 tablespoon olive oil and sauté 2 chopped shallots and 2 crushed garlic cloves for 1–2 minutes for potato gnocchi in a fast tomato sauce. 2 tablespoons white wine, a 400 g (13 oz) diced tomato can, a pinch of dried chili flakes, 2 teaspoons thyme leaves Cook for 5–6 minutes on low heat. Meanwhile, in a saucepan of boiling water, prepare 800 g (134 lb) ready-made gnocchi for 2 minutes. Drain and toss the cooked gnocchi in the tomato sauce, then top with parmesan cheese shavings and serve. Cooking time is 10 minutes total.

Chapter Forty-two

NAAN

grilled naan with coconut dahl

4 servings

10 minutes total cooking time

1 tablespoon oil (vegetable)

1 finely sliced onion

2 tblsp. curry paste (korma)

125 g (4 oz) washed split red lentils

coconut milk, 400 g (13 oz)

peppercorns

fresh coriander, chopped

Breads known as naans

In a heavy-bottomed saucepan, heat the oil and sauté the onion for 1 minute, stirring constantly, before adding the curry paste and lentils.

Fill the can with water and add it to the lentils after pouring in the coconut milk. Cook for 8–9 minutes, uncovered, until the lentils are cooked and the mixture is thick and pulpy. Season with black pepper and coriander leaves, then serve.

Meanwhile, cook the naan breads lightly on a preheated high grill until brown and toasty. Cut the dahl into fingers and serve alongside for dipping.

In a large saucepan, heat 4 tablespoons vegetable oil and cook 1 roughly chopped onion, 1 trimmed and roughly chopped large courgette, and 1 trimmed and roughly chopped aubergine for 10 minutes, stirring periodically, until soft. 4 tablespoons korma curry paste and 125 g (4 oz) rinsed split red lentils, then 600 ml (1 pint) vegetable stock, and cook for 10–15 minutes, until thick and pulpy. Meanwhile, make the toasted naan fingers as directed in the coconut dahl recipe and serve with the dahl. Cooking time is 30 minutes total.

Chapter Forty-three

COURGETTE AND FETA FRITTERS

4 servings

Cooking time total: 20 minutes

1 gently beaten egg

1 oz. self-raising flour (25 g)

buttermilk (about 2 tablespoons)

2 big shredded courgettes

a smidgeon of dill, chopped

3 chopped spring onions

feta cheese, 150 g (5 oz)

olive oil, 75 ml (3 fl oz)

Pita breads, toasted, to serve

Salad with peppers

2 jarred pre-roasted peppers, chopped

a quarter-cup of lemon juice

2 tablespoons extra virgin olive oil

a handful of chopped mint leaves

Combine the egg, flour, and buttermilk in a mixing bowl and whisk until smooth. Place the courgettes in a clean tea towel and wring out any excess water before mixing with the dill and spring onions in the batter. Crumble the feta in a bowl.

In a big nonstick frying pan, heat half of the oil. To make the fritters, pour heaping spoonful of the mixture into the pan and flatten gently with the back of a spoon. Cook for 3 minutes, until golden brown, then flip and cook for another 2 minutes, until golden brown and cooked through. Keep heated by draining on kitchen paper. Using the leftover mixture and oil, repeat the process.

Combine the roasted peppers, lemon juice, oil, and mint in a mixing bowl. Serve with toasted pita breads alongside the fritters.

Slice 2 courgettes into long, thin strips for a zesty couscous, courgette, and feta salad. Rub with 2 tablespoons olive oil and heat for 1 minute on each side on a hot griddle pan until lightly browned. In a mixing dish, combine 300 g (10 oz) couscous and 400 ml (14 fl oz) boiling vegetable stock. Cover and let aside for 5 minutes before adding 4 tablespoons lemon juice, 5 tablespoons olive oil, and a handful of parsley and mint.

Season with salt and pepper, then add the courgettes and 75 g (3 oz) sun-blush tomatoes. 50 g (2 oz) roasted pine nuts and 100 g (312 oz) crumbled feta cheese are sprinkled over the top. Cooking time is 10 minutes total.

Chapter Forty-four

RISOTTO WITH TOMATOES

4 servings

30 minutes total cooking time

1 tablespoon extra virgin olive oil

1 diced onion

2 smashed garlic cloves

Plum tomatoes, 100 g (312 oz)

ready-made tomato sauce, 200 mL (7 fl oz)

12 pint hot vegetable stock (300 mL)

arborio rice, 200 g (7 oz)

Sun-dried tomatoes, sliced into strips, 50 g (2 oz)

2 tblsp basil leaves, shredded

seasoning with salt and pepper

40 g (134 oz) parmesan cheese, grated

In a saucepan, heat the olive oil and sauté the onion and garlic for 5–6 minutes.

Meanwhile, pour boiling water over the tomatoes in a large mixing bowl. Allow 30 seconds to stand before draining and refreshing under cold water. After removing the skins, the tomatoes should be deseeded and chopped.

In a small saucepan, bring the tomato sauce and stock to a simmer.

Continue to mix the rice into the onions for 1–2 minutes, or until the edges of the grains appear transparent.

Stir in a ladle of tomato sauce and stock at a time until it is completely absorbed. Continue adding a ladle of hot stock at a time until the rice is 'al dente.'

Season to taste with the chopped tomatoes, sliced sun-dried tomatoes, and basil.

Serve with grated parmesan cheese on top.

Skin and chop 4 plum tomatoes, as for tomato risotto, and combine with 4 sliced spring onions, 400 g (13 oz) ready-cooked rice, 200 g (7 oz) diced mozzarella cheese, and 2 tablespoons chopped basil leaves in a quick tomato & rice salad. To serve, season with salt and pepper and drizzle with 2 tablespoons olive oil. Cooking time is 10 minutes total.

Chapter Forty-five

CHEESE AND SPINACH CALZONE

4 servings

30 minutes total cooking time

500 g (1 pound) strong bread flour, plus a little more for dusting

1 sachet dried yeast, 7 g (14 oz)

a grain of salt

3 tablespoons extra virgin olive oil

Warm water, 300 mL (12 pint)

Spinach, 300 g (10 oz)

Ricotta cheese, 400 g (13 oz)

4 tblsp parmesan cheese, grated

4 tablespoons pecorino cheese, grated

4 sliced spring onions

1 teaspoon black pepper, freshly ground

To prepare the dough, whisk together the flour, yeast, and salt in a large mixing basin. Create a well in the middle. 1 tablespoon olive oil and the majority of the measured water Mix everything together with your hands, adding extra water as needed to get a soft, but not sticky dough.

Knead the dough for 5–10 minutes on a floured work surface, until it is smooth and elastic. Divide the dough into four equal pieces and roll each into a 20 cm (8 inch) circle.

In a frying pan, heat the remaining olive oil, then add the spinach and cook for 2–3 minutes, or until totally wilted. In a mixing basin, combine the remaining ingredients.

Divide the mixture evenly among the four dough circles, laying it on one half of each circle and leaving a 2.5 cm (1 inch) clean edge. Using water to wipe the edges, fold the other half over the filling and squeeze the sides together to seal. Place the calzones on a baking sheet and bake for 6–8 minutes, until the dough is done and the filling is hot, at 220°C (425°F), gas mark 7.

In a frying pan, heat 1 tablespoon olive oil and sauté 1 sliced red onion for a few minutes before adding 250 g (8 oz) spinach leaves and stirring to wilt. Remove from heat and stir in 4 tablespoons parmesan cheese and 200 g (7 oz) broken mozzarella. 4 pita breads, heated, sliced along one side, and opened up Make a spinach filling in each pita. Cooking time is 10 minutes total.

Tartlets with feta, spring onions, and walnuts

4 servings

10 minutes total cooking time

4 brown bread pieces, crusts removed

150 g (5 oz) crumbled feta cheese

2 finely sliced spring onions

walnut bits, 25 g (1 oz), finely crushed

cut into quarters 8 cherry tomatoes

1 tablespoon extra virgin olive oil

seasoning with salt and pepper

to assist

mixed salad leaves, 200 g (7 oz)

12 sliced cucumbers

Using a rolling pin, thinly roll out the bread. Cut each slice into a circle with a diameter of about 12 cm (5 inches) and push the circles into four large nonstick muffin or yorkshire pudding tins. Cook for 7–8 minutes in a preheated oven at 200°C (400°F), gas mark 6, until crisp and golden.

Meanwhile, combine the crumbled feta, spring onions, walnut bits, and tomatoes in a mixing bowl. Season with salt and pepper, then spoon into the heated tart shells. Serve with a mixed leaf and cucumber salad drizzled with olive oil.

Roll 500 g (1 lb) ready-made puff pastry into a 30 x 20 cm rectangle for the feta, spring onion, and walnut tart (12 x 8 inches). Place on a lightly greased baking sheet and score a border all the way around the pastry, without quite cutting through, about 1.5 cm (34 inch) in from the edges. Within the border, scatter 200 g (7 oz) crumbled feta, 4 thinly sliced spring onions, 50 g (2 oz) walnut pieces, and 12 quartered cherry tomatoes. Drizzle with 1 tablespoon olive oil and bake for about 20 minutes at 200°C (400°F), gas mark 6, until crisp and golden. Serve alongside a salad. Cooking time is 30 minutes total.

Chapter Forty-six

PASTA

from a delicatessen

4 servings

Cooking time total: 20 minutes

Fusilli, 375 g (12 oz)

2 tbsp olive oil (extra virgin)

1 tblsp balsamic vinaigrette

12 teaspoon mustard (dijon)

12 teaspoon honey (clear)

1 smashed garlic clove

10 sliced sun-dried tomatoes

drained and halved 400 g (13 ounce) can artichoke hearts

Parmesan cheese shavings, 100 g (312 oz)

Cook the fusilli for 9–12 minutes in a pot of boiling water, or according to the package directions.

To make the dressing, whisk together the oil, vinegar, mustard, honey, and garlic.

Drain the pasta and combine it with the dressing in the pan. Warm through by stirring in the sun-dried tomatoes and artichoke hearts.

Serve in shallow pasta bowls with parmesan shavings on top.

Slice 2 baguettes into 16 slices and lay on a baking pan for artichoke and sun-dried tomato bruschetta. Toast for 2–3 minutes on each side after drizzling with 2 tablespoons olive oil. Using a peeled garlic clove, rub one side of each slice. A 400 g (13 oz) can artichoke hearts, drained and sliced, and 12 chopped sun-dried tomatoes go on top of the bruschetta. 2 tablespoons toasted pine nuts and tiny basil leaves to garnish Cooking time is 10 minutes total.

Chapter Forty-seven

TAGINE DE LEGUMES

de Maroc

4 servings

30 minutes total cooking time

Couscous, 200 g (7 oz)

boiling water, 550 ml (18 fl oz)

2 tbsp sunflower seed oil

1 big coarsely chopped onion

2 minced garlic cloves

1 teaspoon fresh root ginger, grated

2 tablespoons cumin powder

1 teaspoon coriander powder

2 tablespoons cinnamon powder

1 teaspoon turmeric powder

2 tsp red chili flakes (dry)

1 tablespoon paste de harissa

400 g (13 oz) chopped tomatoes in a can

heated vegetable stock, 250 mL (8 fl oz)

2 red peppers, de-seeded, cored, and sliced into bite-size pieces

700 g (112 lb) peeled, deseeded, and cubed butternut squash

Golden sultanas, 100 g (312 oz)

seasoning with salt and pepper

To garnish, fresh coriander, chopped

Season the couscous with salt in a large heatproof bowl. Pour over the measured water, cover with cling film, and set aside for 10 minutes, or until the water is absorbed, as directed on the package. Separate the grains with a fork, then set aside and keep heated.

Meanwhile, in a large frying pan, heat the oil, add the onion, and sauté for 2–3 minutes, tossing regularly, until softened. Bring the garlic, ginger, ground spices, chili flakes, harissa, tomatoes, and stock to a boil, then lower to a low heat, cover, and cook for 10–12 minutes.

Recover and increase the heat to medium after adding the red peppers, squash, and sultanas. Season to taste after 10–15 minutes of simmering, or until the vegetables are soft.

Serve the couscous in warm dishes with the tagine ladled over it and garnished with chopped coriander.

Cut 2 large courgettes, 2 cored and deseeded red peppers, and 1 eggplant into bits and place in a large mixing bowl for moroccan kebabs. Toss the veggies in a mixture of 8 tablespoons olive oil, 1 tablespoon harissa paste, 2 lemons' juice, and a small handful of chopped coriander. Season the vegetables and thread them onto 12 metal skewers. Cook for 10–12 minutes, flipping once, under a preheated medium grill. Serve alongside couscous. Cooking time is 20 minutes total.

Chapter Forty-eight

PEPPER PIZZA

4 servings

10 minutes total cooking time

a total of four pita breads

ketchup (tomato): 4 tbsp

4 jarred ready-to-eat red and yellow peppers, drained and sliced

4 sliced spring onions

sliced mozzarella cheese, 150 g (5 oz)

Rocket leaves, a small handful

On each side, toast the pita breads for 2 minutes. 1 tablespoon tomato ketchup, roasted peppers, spring onions, and mozzarella

Cook for 4–6 minutes, until bubbling and brown, under a hot grill that has been preheated. Serve with rocket on top.

In a large saucepan, bring 1 litre (134 quarts) water to a boil for the polenta pepper pizza. Slowly pour in 250 g (8 oz) polenta while continuously stirring. Season with 1 teaspoon dry oregano and cook for another 8–10 minutes, stirring constantly, until the polenta is thick. Divide in half, pour onto two lightly oiled baking sheets, and spread into a 12 inch thick circle. Preheat the oven to 200°C (400°F), gas mark 6, and bake for 12 minutes. Cover the polenta with 400 g (13 oz) chopped tomatoes, 350 g (1112 oz) ready-roasted peppers, cut into strips, and 10–12 coarsely broken basil leaves, then 250 g (8 oz) sliced mozzarella cheese. Return to the oven for another 12–15 minutes, or until the cheese is golden and bubbling. Cut into wedges and serve immediately. Cooking time is 40 minutes total.

Chapter Forty-nine

SPAGHETTI

with basil and rocket pesto

4 servings

Cooking time total: 20 minutes

sunflower or pumpkin seeds, 50 g (2 oz)

Wholewheat spaghetti, 500 g (1 lb)

1 clove garlic, coarsely chopped

1 tiny basil bunch

Rocket leaves, 75 g (3 oz)

25 g (1 oz) finely grated parmesan cheese, with enough to serve (optional)

6 tablespoons extra virgin olive oil

a quarter-cup of lemon juice

seasoned with salt & pepper

In a small dry frying pan, roast the seeds for 3–4 minutes, stirring the pan often, until lightly toasted and brown. Allow to cool on a platter.

Cook the spaghetti in a large saucepan of lightly salted boiling water for 11–12 minutes, or until 'al dente,' or according to the package directions.

Meanwhile, using a pestle and mortar, pound the garlic with a liberal teaspoon of sea salt. Pound in the basil and rocket leaves until a coarse pulp forms.

To make a paste, pound the toasted seeds, then transfer to a bowl with the cheese, olive oil, and lemon juice. Season to taste with a generous amount of black pepper and, if necessary, additional salt.

Drain the pasta and combine it with the pesto right away. Serve in 4 shallow bowls with more cheese on top, if preferred.

Cook 500 g (1 lb) ready-made gnocchi in a large pot of gently salted boiling water for about 2 minutes, or until just soft, according to package instructions, for creamy gnocchi pesto bake. In the meantime, combine 4 tablespoons ready-made green pesto and 300 mL (12 pint) crème fraîche in a mixing bowl. Add the cooked gnocchi and 2 tablespoons grated parmesan cheese, then transfer to a large ovenproof dish. Cook for 20 minutes at 190°C (375°F), gas mark 5 in a preheated oven until bubbling and brown. If desired, top with additional rocket leaves. Cooking time is 30 minutes total.

Chapter Fifty

ARRABBIATA

Arrabbiata dip with polenta chips

2 people

10 minutes total cooking time

ready-made polenta, 500 g (1 lb)

3 tbsp. ordinary flour (for dusting)

4 tablespoons extra virgin olive oil

375 g (12 oz) store-bought arrabbiata pasta sauce in a carton

to assist

Leaves of the rocket

shavings of parmesan cheese

Shake off the excess flour after cutting the polenta block into chip-shaped fingers.

In a frying pan, heat the oil and cook the polenta chips for 2–3 minutes on each side over medium-high heat, until crisp and golden. Keep heated by draining on kitchen paper.

In a separate skillet, heat the arrabbiata sauce. Serve with the polenta chips, rocket leaves, and parmesan shavings in small dishes.

Pour half a 375 g (12 oz) carton arrabbiata sauce onto the bottom of a medium ovenproof dish for arrabbiata polenta bake. Top the sauce with 300 g (10 oz) sliced polenta, 50 g (2 oz) diced mozzarella, and 2 tablespoons grated parmesan cheese. Pour the remaining sauce over the top and sprinkle with 75 g (3 oz) chopped mozzarella and 2 tablespoons grated parmesan cheese. Preheat oven to 220°C (425°F), gas mark 7, and bake for 20–25 minutes, or until brown and bubbly. As with polenta chips with arrabbiata dip, serve with a salad. Cooking time is 30 minutes total.

Chapter Fifty-one

MEDITERRANEAN BEANS

4 servings

10 minutes total cooking time

2 tbsp olive oil (extra virgin)

1 diced red onion

1 smashed garlic clove

12 tbsp cumin seeds

400 g (13 oz) rinsed and drained cannellini beans

75 g (3 oz) quartered cherry tomatoes

2 tablespoons sage, chopped

4 crusty bread slices

seasoning with salt and pepper

To serve, 25 g (1 oz) grated manchego cheese

In a large frying pan, heat the oil, then add the onion and sauté for 1–2 minutes. Cook for another 2–3 minutes after adding the garlic and cumin seeds.

Add the beans and stir to combine, allowing them to absorb the flavors before adding the tomatoes. Season with salt and pepper and heat through the sage.

Meanwhile, toast the bread for 2–3 minutes on each side under a hot grill that has been warmed. Serve with a dollop of sour cream and a sprinkling of cheese on top.

In a big frying pan, heat 1 tablespoon olive oil, add 1 large chopped onion and 2 crushed garlic cloves, and gently cook for 5 minutes until softened, for mixed bean goulash. Cook for another 3–4 minutes after adding 100 g (312 oz) chopped chestnut mushrooms. Cook for another 1–2 minutes after adding 1 tablespoon smoked paprika. Add a 400 g (13 oz) chopped tomato can, 200 ml (7 fl oz) hot vegetable stock, and a 400 g (13 ounce) washed and drained can of mixed beans. Bring to a boil, then lower to a low heat and continue to cook for 12–14 minutes, or until the sauce is thick and glossy. Serve with cooked rice and, if desired, soured cream dollops. Cooking time is 30 minutes total.

Chapter Fifty-two

GRATIN

gratin with butternut squash and broccoli

4 servings

Cooking time total: 20 minutes

Purple sprouting broccoli, 200 g (7 oz), trimmed

300 g (10 oz) peeled, deseeded, and diced butternut squash

200 g (7 oz) halved mushrooms

60 g butter (214 oz)

2 tablespoons all-purpose flour

milk, 400 mL (14 fl oz)

2 teaspoons mustard (whole grain)

100 g (312 oz) grated cheddar cheese

In a steamer, cook the vegetables for 8–10 minutes, or until tender.

In a small pot, melt the butter, then mix in the flour to produce a roux. Cook for 1–2 minutes, then whisk in the milk gradually and continue to cook, stirring constantly, until the sauce is thick and smooth. Combine the mustard and half of the shredded cheese in a mixing bowl.

Pour the sauce over the veggies in an ovenproof dish and top with the remaining cheese. Cook for 5–6 minutes under a preheated hot grill, until bubbling and brown.

Cook 400 g (13 oz) peeled, deseeded, and diced butternut squash and 150 g (5 oz) peeled and diced potatoes in a saucepan of boiling water for 8 minutes until cooked, for cheesy butternut mash with broccoli and poached eggs. In the meantime, heat a saucepan of water to a gentle simmer and swirl it with a large spoon. Cook for 3 minutes after cracking two eggs into the water. Keep heated by removing with a slotted spoon. Repeat with the remaining two eggs. Steam 400 g (13 oz) broccoli florets in a separate pan until soft. Drain the squash and potatoes and mix with 75 g (3 oz) shredded cheddar cheese in the pan. Serve with 2 tablespoons grated parmesan cheese on top of the broccoli and poached eggs. Cooking time is 10 minutes total.

CPSIA information can be obtained
at www.ICGtesting.com
Printed in the USA
LVHW060214160722
723616LV00015B/754

9 781804 769010